AS YOU READ THESE PAGES
IT WILL HELP YOU TO LEARN ABOUT
HEALTHY AND HAPPY LIVING
WITH DIABETES . . .

Hi, Sugar!

Hi, Sugar!

by Vivian G. Lessel

A Friendly Patient to Patient Chat

about Diabetes

B & B PUBLISHING HOUSE

Tucson, Arizona

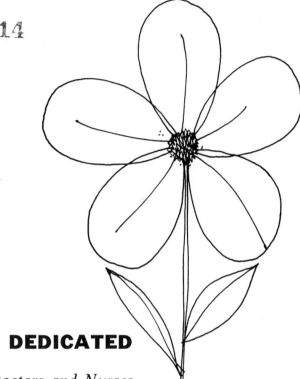

DEDICATED

to all Doctors and Nurses
Technicians and Scientists
who devote their lives

to

Preserving Life

and

Creating Happiness

for

Diabetics Everywhere

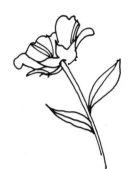

INTRODUCTION

"Hi, Sugar!" was written for diabetic patients—and their families by a woman who had diabetes for 36 years. She was a housewife and secretary, who spoke out of a knowledge and experience with diabetes that was impressive. She understood the need people have, of philosophically accepting their condition, once it is discovered.

She appreciated the importance of their taking daily injections of insulin when their physicians advise them to take it. She knew it is of utmost importance to exercise care in the day to day control and management of diabetes. These are highly desirable goals that physicians want their diabetic patients to achieve.

Reading "Hi, Sugar!" can help diabetics to achieve these goals, for the book has great merit. It is useful to those who suddenly find themselves in need of reading and knowing about diabetes and its successful control.

It is not intended to be a manual for self care; indeed, the author makes it very clear that diabetic patients need to see their physicians regularly for counsel and the periodic adjustments in the management of their diabetes.

L. P. HOWELL, M.D.
Rochester, Minnesota

A DOCTOR'S PRESCRIPTION

The patient and physician must know each other very well. Vivian Lessel and I were friendly during our physician-patient relationship. She would bring copious notes to my office with her so that we might discuss each phase of her illness.

A patient must exercise strict personal discipline. Diabetes is not a game, but must be considered a very serious condition at all times, regardless of how well the patient feels subjectively.

A diabetic must cooperate with his physician. He must not experiment with diet or medications.

A diabetic patient must have a guide. This book (or any other) will be of value only, if followed closely.

The physician must prescribe reading for the patient, in addition to diet and medications. A layman's book such as this one is easy to understand. In this volume Mrs. Lessel has shown the intense understanding she had for her illness. She adopted a practical, sensible attitude, and did not feel that diabetes was a curse. This alone should serve to encourage her readers.

I prescribe the reading of this book by the diabetic and his social circle as a help to happy and healthy diabetic living.

I further hope that each reader will enjoy it as much as I have.

JOSEPH C. KING, M.D.
Chicago, Illinois

A LEGACY TO DIABETICS

Vivian Lessel has written HI, SUGAR! for the diabetic in terms easily understood by the layman. She speaks from long-standing experience about a disease nearly as complex as life itself.

She was indeed a remarkable woman. She learned during her more than 35 years with diabetes mellitus, that a diabetic must try to know as much as possible about his disease in order for him to control it well.

He must follow instructions meticulously and be willing to appraise his physician of all his problems—emotional as well as physical—and seek competent advice whenever he has a question about medication, diet or any other aspect of daily living.

Her goal was always to help her fellow diabetic and thereby she helped herself.

In this book, Mrs. Lessel discusses many of the difficult situations which confront the diabetic and explains how each can be approached calmly and rationally. She has liberally sprinkled the book with light poetry which reveals the true nature of the authoress and makes reading it a delightful experience.

The book is extremely well written, factual and complete and is a worthwhile addition to every diabetic's library.

Thank you for caring enough to write HI, SUGAR! and leaving it as a legacy to ALL diabetics.

HAROLD W. KOHL, JR., M.D.
Tucson, Arizona

ACKNOWLEDGMENTS

THE AMERICAN DIABETES ASSOCIATION,
New York City. Statistical information.

THE AMERICAN MEDICAL ASSOCIATION,
Chicago, Illinois. Information on identification.

Illustrations and Cover designed by
Richard W. Mlodock

PREFACE

Diabetes Is Serious
Diabetes Is for Keeps
Diabetes Is Not a Dread Disease, because—
Diabetes Is Controllable

Written in the memory of many today, is the time when the diagnosis of diabetes usually meant an early death.

With the discovery of insulin in 1921, the diabetic was reprieved from this sentence. The impact of this liberation is not yet completely understood.

Today, the condition itself is just as severe, and when UNcontrolled, the results are just as devastating. However, the controlled diabetic, through insulin and diet, has been able to change his life, from one of doom to one of deliverance.

In 1928, when insulin was entrusted to diabetics for self-administration at home, a great deal of responsibility went with it. There is perhaps no other illness which requires so much from the patient, as does diabetes.

The approaches to this responsibility of diabetic living are manyfold, but a complete diabetic education is the ONLY basis for intelligent living and control.

Diabetics are eager to learn what they can about the treatment of their diabetes. They know that to live successfully with this condition, takes great courage, self-denial and self-control. Although, the diabetic's life may not always be easy, victory can be his reward.

The author has sought to present facts and suggestions, experienced and observed, for successful diabetic living.

If YOU are the diabetic, be a member of the family with a happy heart, learn to understand the importance of good control and its application, thereby, not only helping yourself, but also those who are walking with you.

If you are NOT the diabetic, endeavor to become helpful to those who are. This can be done through a cooperative spirit, based on understanding.

May ALL who read this book, be helped to learn about the diabetic's lifelong companion—diabetes itself.

*   *   *   *   *   *   *   *

The name "Jolene Jordan" is used as a fictitious name for the author.

—V.G.L.

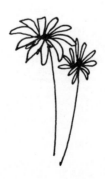

Jolene's husband wants to add this tribute:

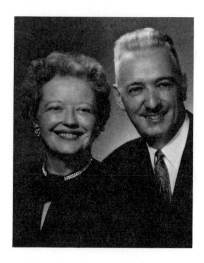

Shortly after completing her manuscript, God called Jolene home to be with Him.

Her efforts to put together her diabetic experiences, observations and information, were motivated by a sincere desire to help ALL diabetics live happily each day and hour.

As her husband, I know that she not only tried, but succeeded beautifully, to live her own life happily, each day and hour.

Yes—even to the last minute.

It is because of her beautiful life that I, her husband, want to add her real name:

VIVIAN GERTRUDE LESSEL to HER list of dedicatees.

—W.M.L.

TABLE OF CONTENTS

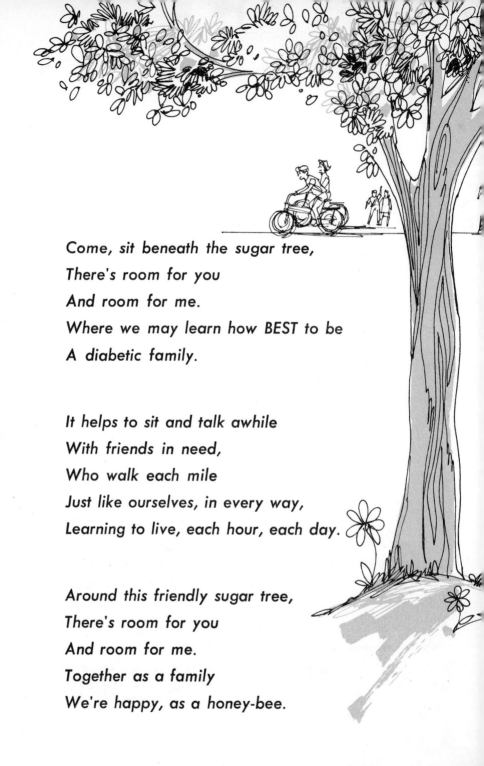

Come, sit beneath the sugar tree,
There's room for you
And room for me.
Where we may learn how BEST to be
A diabetic family.

It helps to sit and talk awhile
With friends in need,
Who walk each mile
Just like ourselves, in every way,
Learning to live, each hour, each day.

Around this friendly sugar tree,
There's room for you
And room for me.
Together as a family
We're happy, as a honey-bee.

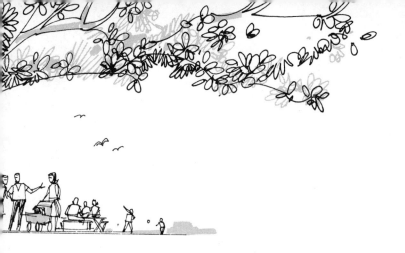

SUGAR TALK

There are an estimated 200 million diabetics in the world. This is a large family of folk, united with a feeling of friendship, because they are interlocked with identical problems and solutions.

After the medical basics for diabetic control, taught by the doctor, are understood and applied, the diabetic is ready to adjust his life to everyday living. He is anxious to find the best way this may be done.

Each diabetic must realize the seriousness of his illness, and accept the fact that it is for keeps. He must secure a complete knowledge of symptoms and treatment for successful diabetic living.

Many years ago, Hedda Hopper was describing in her newspaper column, a young woman who had been enjoying an unusually successful career, and fell victim to diabetes. Her column read, "She was catapulted into a bottomless pit!"

Prior to the use of insulin, a diabetic, undetected, untreated, or uncontrolled, was, we might very well say, catapulted.

In "the bottomless pit" the patient may find blindness, gangrene, heart trouble, rapid hardening of the arteries, liver complications, deterioration of the nervous system and—death. A grim picture.

Today, we have a bright horizon in the miracle medicine—INSULIN!

This bright horizon has illuminated the path of the diabetic for the last 50 years. After the discovery of insulin, it took at least ten years of experimentation, education of patients, their families and the general public, to make insulin acceptable, as the only adequate treatment for diabetes.

When Jolene Jordan's doctor discovered her diabetes in 1932, a relative wrote, "Don't let them start shooting that new medicine into you. If you do, you will NEVER recover from diabetes. I know for a fact, you can control diabetes ONLY with food. If you start taking insulin, you will always have to take it."

No doubt this same message went out to thousands of diabetic patients for many years, and it was against these untruths and opinions, that doctors struggled.

Some of these fallacies are still present today, and the time is long overdue, that this image be wiped out.

If YOU are an unknown PREdiabetic, or if you know you have sugar in the urine and are not seeking your doctor's help, or not using the knowledge you have already received from him, then you too may expect to be "catapulted."

When one is told for the first time that he has diabetes, or when a member of the family or a friend, becomes diabetic, very often the first question asked, is "What is diabetes?"

Diabetes occurs when the insulin producing cells of the pancreas, fail to function, varying from partial to complete failure. Insulin from the pancreas is needed to turn the carbohydrates (sugars and starches) we eat, into energy and heat for the body.

When the pancreas fails to do its part in the digestive system, sugar accumulates in the blood and the individual becomes diabetic. The pancreas of a diabetic, already lazy, may watch as the food is swallowed, fall back (in consternation) on a soft bed of intestines, and go to sleep. Here then, the diabetic is born!

However, the insulin the pancreas fails to produce, is "substituted for" by the injection of animal insulin, which fortunately, works in the human body.

The CAUSE of diabetes is not yet known. Science has been searching for many years, but success has not yet come. Research is exploring new approaches constantly, trying to discover the cause of this gland failure.

The SYMPTOMS of diabetes may appear gradually. It is even possible to have mild diabetes for many years, without ANY symptoms. When the condition progresses, symptoms begin to appear, such as extreme thirst and excessive urination.

These two symptoms are considered by many, to be primary. Others are, weakness to the point of exhaustion, increased appetite, a rapid "gain" in weight which suddenly may reverse itself to a rapid "loss" of weight.

Related symptoms may be severe itching of the skin, frequent boils, open wounds slow or refusing to heal, blurring of vision and slow recovery from minor illnesses.

Jolene Jordan, well recalls her own weakness, which was almost nauseous. She was so weak, in fact, that one day, when the dry cleaner called to pick up her husband's coat, she couldn't carry it to the door, nor could she find strength to remove the handkerchiefs and gloves from the pockets. When the honest cleaner returned them later, she could scarcely find the energy to open the door.

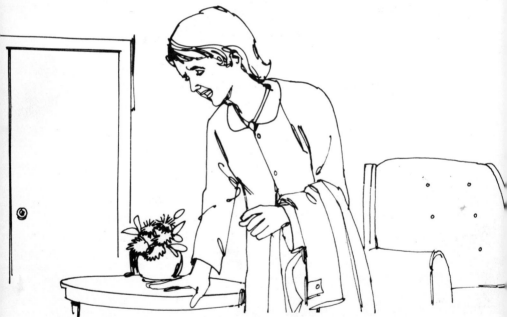

Her thirst was overpowering. She recalls, on many occasions, after drinking eight to ten glasses of water, that her throat stuck together like flypaper, and her mouth felt like it was filled with balls of cotton.

The onset of diabetes is not always the same. Some patients notice only the weakness, others only the thirst. Some may notice only the itching of the skin, while others may say, "I'm just too lazy for words."

It has been proved that diabetes is hereditary. Some families may produce many diabetics, while others produce none. Diabetes does not announce its approach, but comes silently and unexpectedly.

The early stages are often overlooked because the victim has not been alerted to its possible arrival. Its advances are slow, and by the time the symptoms force him to the doctor, it is often too late to prescribe a simple control.

Until the discovery of insulin, there was "no control" except through restriction of food. The severity of the case, determined the length of life, that remained for the patient.

Since 1921, many varieties of the liquid insulin, and several varieties of blood-sugar-lowering-pills and capsules, have been discovered.

So successful has been the use of insulin, or the use of oral products, that together with controlled food intake and adequate exercise, the life expectancy of the diabetic has been extended to include all of the normal activities of the NON-diabetic.

There are five classifications of diabetics:

> *The Prediabetic (the unknown)*
> *The New Diabetic*
> *The Mild Diabetic*
> *The Child Diabetic*
> *The Complicated (brittle) Diabetic*

The patient in each of these categories, must have a working knowledge of adequate control. A simple program of education for the millions of people around the world, both diabetic and non-diabetic, may be helpful.

A recent survey of 1,800 diabetics, on the question of whether or not they understood their diets, and if they followed them, revealed some appalling results.

ONLY 10 PERCENT OF THOSE QUESTIONED, KNEW WHAT THEIR DIET AND SCHEDULE WAS ALL ABOUT! 24 percent said, they did not follow the diet. Their negligence was not willful, but a result of not having understood their needs. Because they did not understand, they skipped it altogether. This can be fatal.

The lack of knowledge among diabetic patients, concerning their illness, is frightening. A diabetic woman recently wrote a doctor that she had been a diabetic for a year and was taking insulin. She had heard the word carbohydrates, but did not know its meaning.

This makes an informed diabetic cringe, for if all of this woman's diabetic education was as limited as her question would indicate, there is room for alarm.

Diabetics are dealing with a treacherous and temperamental foe, which doesn't allow too much time for making mistakes. Education regarding this illness is a "must."

While the word "diabetes" may have been heard by many, a close-up view or a personal experience with it, may have never occurred.

Every member of the diabetic's family, his friends, his co-workers and yes, the public service personnel, all need a general diabetic education. Each one will then be prepared to extend intelligent help to the diabetic, should he need it.

Diabetic education is also important to all NON-diabetics. Statistics show that many so-called non-diabetics are actually "potential prediabetics." If EVERYONE WERE AWARE OF THIS THREAT TO HIS HEALTH, HE WOULD IMMEDIATELY SEEK COMPLETE INFORMATION FROM HIS DOCTOR.

Also, the non-diabetic, with a diabetic education, may be helpful in discovering a prediabetic in his own family.

YES, EVERYONE NEEDS TO UNDERSTAND THIS "SUGAR TALK," AND FIND HIS PLACE IN THE WORLD OF DIABETIC LIVING!

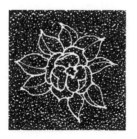

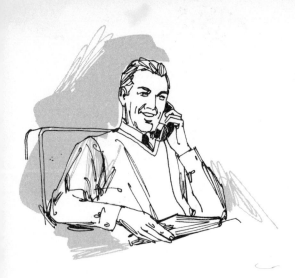

When the doctor says, you're diabetic,
And you don't know what to do,
About the many little things,
That are happening to you.

Just call him on the telephone,
If it's urgent, through the day,
Or—wait until you see him next,
To help you, all the way.

You will need him more than you may think,
To gain your strength and vim.
But thru HIS help, you'll feel just fine,
So—confide it ALL in him.

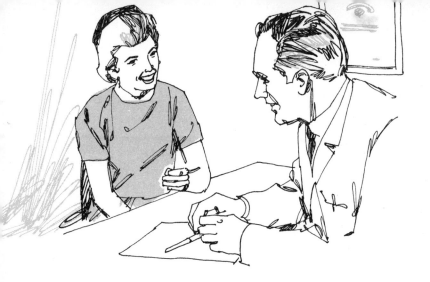

WHEN THE DOCTOR SAYS...

Because the onset of diabetes is gradual and subtle, it is easy to overlook the symptoms, when they begin to appear. This usually delays the visit to the doctor. Much valuable time is lost, because diabetes does not stand still.

When the first symptom does appear, which may be an exhausting weakness, many patients have been known to resort to tonics and other "blood building" remedies. This does not help, and their condition only worsens. By the time they are forced to seek the doctor's help, the illness may have progressed to a more serious stage.

Had the doctor been given the opportunity to diagnose the problems in the first place, the illness might have been controlled with diet, or with one of the oral compounds.

When the visit is delayed, it may be necessary to control the sugar with daily injections of insulin.

Each diabetic is an individual, and therefore, different. Diabetics vary in intensity of the illness, in age, in needs, in symptoms, and as a result, vary in the prescribed treatment. These are some of the reasons why the doctor is the ONLY ONE who can authoritatively say, "You are a diabetic," and only he can prescribe the treatment.

Neither an Aunt Flo, who may be an excellent nurse, nor a neighbor, who may be a well-controlled diabetic of long standing, is qualified to diagnose the symptoms.

TRAINING CENTERS

If the diabetes is questionable or complicated, the family doctor may, of his own volition, suggest that the patient visit a large clinic, or a specialist in internal medicine, because he values the diagnostic opinion and training program of such a clinic or specialist.

If a visit is possible, it may prove quite beneficial to the patient and to the family physician as well.

Clinics are organized as training centers, and the specialist has an organized program for training, to assist the family doctor. It is much easier, for the family physician to treat a knowledgeable patient.

The clinic and the specialist will forward their findings and recommendations to the family doctor, who will pursue the daily treatment of the diabetes and take care of any other complication, which may appear.

Thus, the importance of a good family doctor grows, and he becomes the diabetic's best friend.

Among the many phases of the condition, in which the patient must be educated, are types of insulin, reading the syringe properly, drawing the insulin into the syringe, injecting the insulin, learning about food values, the calculated diet, the use of exchange lists, how to make tests accurately, the care of the skin and feet, how to keep daily records, and many more important aspects.

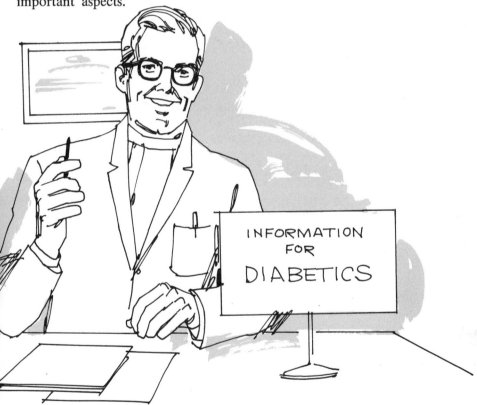

One day, when Jolene was feeling especially appreciative of the help she was receiving, she mentioned to her doctor how much each diabetic relies on the advice of his doctor. He jokingly smiled, "You mean you can't escape us." No, nor would a diabetic want to.

A doctor with the right answers in an emergency, is as close as the phone. For routine questions, he will be happy to help on the next office visit. What more can one ask?

While the doctor is willing and anxious to help, the complications of diabetes are sometimes so involved, that the patient must learn to recognize these problems himself, and know what to do.

Diabetes demands that the doctor and the patient work together, but a large portion of the total responsibility does lie in the hands of the patient.

Even if the doctor were to live in the same home with the patient, or the diabetic found his way, daily, to the doorstep of the doctor, there would still be many decisions which only the patient can make.

The doctor uses his medical knowledge to guide and suggest. The patient uses his doctor's suggestions and the testing results, as the guide-line for his control.

Dr. Russell M. Wilder, for many years a beloved and dedicated doctor for diabetics at Mayo Clinic, had a pet phrase, coupled with his famous smile, "I never break up a winning combination." He instilled confidence within every diabetic. A conscientious and understanding doctor is priceless, and the best reward a patient can give him, is complete cooperation and a "fully controlled" diabetic life. The diabetic must always have a complete understanding of his condition and a willingness to follow the doctor's guidance. Then, and only then, can the doctor and the patient become a winning team.

Should it be necessary, for the diabetic to move to some distant location, he will need to find a new doctor. The present physician, if he is acquainted in the new area, may be able to recommend someone. If not, the patient should seek guidance from other dependable sources such as the state or county Medical Society, and settle the choice BEFORE an illness or problem strikes.

The records from the previous physician will be extremely helpful, and doctors are happy to supply these records, upon request.

Diabetes is only one of a great many illnesses, and the doctors who have chosen to include diabetes in their practice, are the best doctors in the world, to work with diabetics.

This is extremely important, for the happiness of both, the doctor and the patient, is at stake.

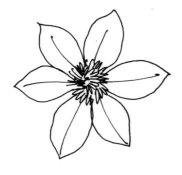

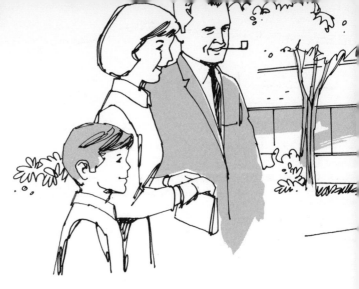

THE DIABETIC FAMILY

We do not know, who next may be
A member of this family.
Make sure of this, in checking through
That you'll find out, BEFORE you too,
Develop symptoms—weakness, thirst.
With health impaired—your bubbles burst.

But should your diabetes show,
Your DOCTOR is the man to know.
So call and see him right away
Please do not wait, do not delay.
He'll help you, how to live and be
A happy member, of this family.

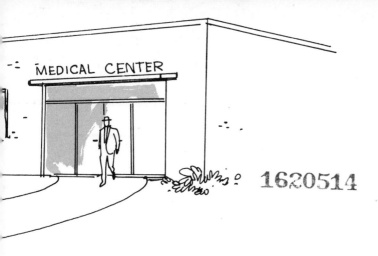

MEDICAL CENTER

1620514

THE PREDIABETIC

Anyone may be a prediabetic. As a rule, the prediabetic has inherited the weakness for diabetes from a long line of diabetic ancestors.

Today, when someone is diagnosed as diabetic, he may say, we have no one in our family who is diabetic. If the records of the illnesses of a diabetic's ancestors could be read today, in the light of present-day medical knowledge, many of them would be found to be diabetic.

Prior to the discovery of insulin, and for many years afterwards, adequate tests to determine the absolute cause of death, were not known. Frequently, heart trouble, brain hemorrhage and other illnesses were blamed, when actually the patient was a diabetic victim.

There are many stages and degrees of diabetic development, and no one knows when, and to whom, this may happen. The prediabetic is the UNKNOWN diabetic.

Although diabetes is thought of as an adult illness, children are known to have been born with it. It has only been in the last few years, that newborn infants of parents who come from a family (or families) with a diabetic history, are tested immediately for sugar in the urine.

This early stage of unknown prediabetics, can be one of the most critical stages of the illness. If not detected, it may develop into a full-blown case of diabetes.

It is the opinion of many leading diabetic doctors, that all diabetics are born as potential prediabetics. They are born with a sluggish pancreas, and depending upon the extent of this sluggishness, the victim may develop the illness at whatever time in life, the insulin producing cells of the pancreas, decide they can work no more.

It is estimated, that for every four known diabetics, there are three unknown. If diabetes is detected BEFORE the symptoms of advanced diabetes reveal themselves, then that person is indeed fortunate. The doctor may indicate that it is possible, for the newly detected diabetic, to control his blood sugar with diet alone.

No insulin injection! Not even pills or capsules to swallow! The "advanced" diabetic, may ask, "How fortunate can a diabetic be?"

It is precisely for the unknown prediabetics that the sound of alarm goes out every November, known as Diabetes Detection Week, sponsored by the American Diabetes Association.

One week before Thanksgiving week, qualified centers are set up all over the country, principally in hospitals, for all those interested in a free urinalysis for sugar. They are asked to bring a small bottle of urine for testing. What could be more simple than that, to detect early symptoms?

Because NO ONE knows for sure, whether diabetes has been in his family or not, everyone SHOULD be tested, at least once a year. If a known diabetic is in the family, then every member of that family (right down through all the cousins), should be tested every three to six months.

Diabetes is sly and comes like a thief in the night. Don't be caught napping.

Sometimes, the known diabetics, are the best people in the world to crusade for detection of prediabetics, because they fully understand, what is at stake. Each could teach his own household to make the test. It is very simple.

The unknown diabetic may delay seeing his doctor, saying, "When spring comes, I'll feel better" or "It's the hot weather, when cooler weather comes, I'll be okay."

The weeks may drag on slowly and the seasons may change, but the condition will not improve. Finally, he is forced to see his doctor.

EARLY TESTING

It is not always easy for the doctor to diagnose an elevated blood sugar. One of the early symptoms of progressing diabetes is weakness, and this could come from many other causes.

The first check the doctor will make is for sugar in the urine, and this test could show "sugar-free."

The doctor knows the prediabetic could have a sugar-free urine, but an elevated blood sugar. So, a blood specimen is taken, at a time scheduled by the doctor.

The test is run immediately and if an elevation in sugar is noted, a drink of high sugar content, usually resembling a malted milk, is given the patient.

When the doctor feels adequate time has elapsed, another blood specimen is taken and tested. If the rise in the blood sugar is abnormal, he feels he has discovered another diabetic. Before arriving at a final decision, however, he may run two or three more tests at a later time, to be positive.

These tests are known as sugar tolerance tests, or as some people like to call them, the diabetic sobriety test.

This test is important to patients with a family history of diabetes. If YOU are a member of a diabetic family, be sure to tell your doctor, as he may want to give you the sugar tolerance test, in addition to the urine test. Doctors tell us, this is the only sure way of discovering a prediabetic.

A young man of 17 was recently discovered to have diabetes, through this method. Because his case had not yet progressed too far, he was able to control the blood sugar with one of the oral preparations, taken before each meal. If he stays closely to the control set up for him, he can always be thankful for the tests given by an alert and knowledgeable doctor.

The question has been asked over and over again, is it possible for a diabetic to be cured of diabetes?

No, not yet. Doctors tell us, that sometimes potential or pre-diabetics, show symptoms resembling diabetes. This may be due to a gain of weight, special stress or some illness.

When these conditions are corrected, the symptoms may disappear, because the sugar in the blood and urine have returned to normal.

However, an alerted prediabetic should always be careful about his food consumption and weight. He should also remember to take frequent urine tests.

A POTENTIAL PREDIABETIC MUST NEVER FALL INTO A FALSE SENSE OF SECURITY!

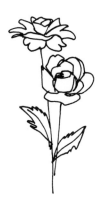

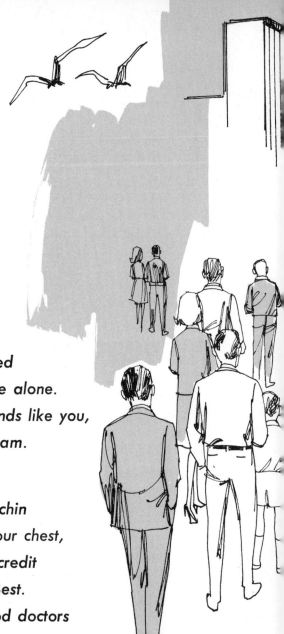

Don't be dismayed
And feel, you are alone.
There are thousands like you,
Wherever you roam.

So UP with your chin
And OUT with your chest,
You MUST be a credit
To Banting and Best.
And ALL the good doctors
Who conscientiously give,
Their talents and time
That diabetics may live.

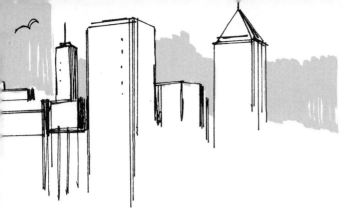

THE NEW DIABETIC

There is a "D" (Discovery) Day for every diabetic. On that day, he may understand the chill, the woman-fisherman felt, who used frozen frogs for bait, and upon reaching into the sack, found they had thawed.

Each diabetic, on his "D" Day, suddenly and surely has felt, what he thought to be, a noose slip about his neck, and realized, it was do or die.

These words portray an ominous feeling, and each one must face his problems squarely. It is only as the diabetic is willing to accept his illness that he can be trained to be a controlled and happy diabetic, and not until then.

When the diabetic has passed the "potential" or "prediabetic" stage, and has been told by his doctor, "You are a full-fledged diabetic," it is then high time for him to face these facts.

He must always keep in close touch with his doctor.
He needs constant treatment, and must learn everything
he can about the administration of it.
He must understand that diabetics eat to live, not live to
eat.   Diabetes is for keeps.

Acceptance of these facts, makes control possible. Only the diabetic himself can decide which road to travel, the one of self-discipline and control, or the other of lackadaisical attitude, with practically no control.

We already know that "education" of the diabetic is essential. He cannot say, "I think this is right" or "I think this is what the doctor said." He must KNOW beyond the shadow of a doubt. He must know how to control his sugar whether by diet, insulin injections or an oral compound, and how to maintain that control 24 hours a day.

Inasmuch as complications can upset the control so quickly, the choice of staying with the correct schedule, as prescribed by the doctor, is the only wise one.

Jolene Jordan made this wise decision many years ago. Her diabetes was complicated, necessitating a tight control, day after day. As she looked back over the many additional complications from which she had been spared, she realized, "It was worth every effort!"

It is true, the new diabetic must learn how to live all over again. When the first restrictions of foods are felt, the first injection of insulin taken, the initial "dropping out" of a few of the activities experienced, then his first thought might be, "Why, oh, why, must this happen to me? It is too hard to live with, why should it be ME?" This is a very human reaction, but it will get you nowhere.

The diabetic cannot waste his time on self-pity. He must accept the facts of his condition, and come to grips with them and win. When this hurdle has been overcome, he is ready to learn how to live with his diabetes.

Someone has said, all men have two vulnerable spots, the stomach and the pocketbook. The new diabetic feels strongly about the first, his stomach. *It isn't what is put into the stomach that causes diabetes, but what we keep out of it, that helps to control it.*

Some new diabetics rebel against this, and this is understandable. Let's face it. One of the greatest pleasures of mankind is the food he chews, savors and drops into that little round pouch that keeps him going from day to day. Just to look at good food starts the salivary glands to flutter, and saliva rushing into the mouth, ready for mastication.

A diabetic's stomach is just as demanding, just as human. He longs for good food. He drools at the thought of good food, and before he learns to control his appetite and food intake, he may "snitch" some food. It isn't long, however, until he learns only to ADMIRE the food he cannot have, and is able to resist the temptation. Sometimes, the stomach seems to know, it is being cheated and rebels, and sends up spasmodic messages for more food, not knowing his little brother, the pancreas, is lying down on the job.

Recently, a young intern was heard to make a cold remark about diabetics who have difficulty staying on their diets. An older and experienced doctor asked, "Have you ever tried to live for just one week on a calculated diet?" The answer was a sheepish, "No." "You should try it sometime," replied the doctor.

It is true, sticking to a calculated diet is certainly not the easiest thing in the world, but the diabetic has discovered that his sense of well-being increases greatly when he adheres to the prescribed diet, and in addition to that, he discovers that this "must" food has become the "best" food in the world.

In the early days of Jolene Jordan's diabetic experience, she fell into coma and was taken to the hospital. Many had doubts she would ever return home.

She was very fortunate that an intern who had been trained at the University of Toronto, by none other than Dr. Charles H. Best, discoverer of insulin, was on hand to treat her.

About three days after her arrival, the intern who had traveled with her through the "dark days," was standing in her room. Suddenly a friend with eyes aglow, and who knew no more about diabetes than Jolene, entered the room bearing a huge luscious cake. It would be impossible to ever forget the expression on the intern's face, and his startled, unbelieving eyes, as he stammered, "A cake, a cake! For YOU?"

Jolene had learned enough, in those few days of hospitalization, to know that cake was certainly not included in her diet, and quickly said assuringly, "Don't worry, you and the nurses may have it, and I'll be happy just to know you are enjoying it." He relaxed and forced a smile, but it did take him several days to recover from the shock. Today, perhaps he too can chuckle over it.

Several years ago, a young woman conducting a research study on diabetes, asked Jolene how long she had known she had diabetes. At that time, it was 19 years. "Well," said the researcher, "then you would have the answer to this one. How long did it take you to ACCEPT diabetes?"

Jolene thought a moment, and said, "Oh, I don't know. I guess right away."

The young woman smiled through her sophisticated approach, and said, "I doubt that very much."

Jolene also smiled and said, "It is true."

The researcher replied, "No one can make such a drastic change in daily living, as a diabetic is called upon to make, and accept it at once."

Jolene pondered these words many times, and still had not made up her mind who was right, probably both.

It is true, the many details we must learn to accept, unfold slowly through the years, but the willingness to accept them, had better come early, or we may not be around later, to make the choice.

While diabetics need exercise for a healthy life, they also require a little more rest than others, in order to maintain energy for their activities.

Recently a woman said, "My diabetic husband seems to need extra sleep. Is this natural or is he ill?"

The answer was, "Diabetics do seem to require more sleep than most people. However, drowsiness is one symptom of uncontrolled diabetes, so be sure his sugar is under control. It would also be wise to make another visit to his doctor, in order to check further on this condition."

Being a NEW diabetic is not easy, but it must become a challenge. There are many adjustments to make and many new things to learn.

Fear Not That Your Life May Come to an End,
For You, the New Diabetic, It Has Just Begun.

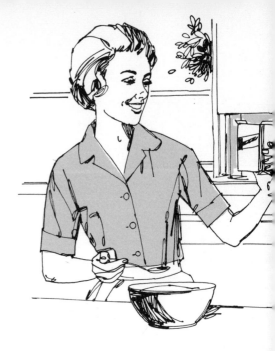

My doctor says, your diabetes
Is as mild as it can be.
And though I take some insulin,
From worry, I am free.

There are no HIGHS, and only LOWS,
In all the tests I make.
My doctor says, "That's very good!"
So I think—I'll bake a cake.

That cake, was one-great-big-mistake,
It was as wrong as it could be.
I've learned my lesson, once again,
For the sugar, shot to three.
        (Actually it was four, but it didn't rhyme.)

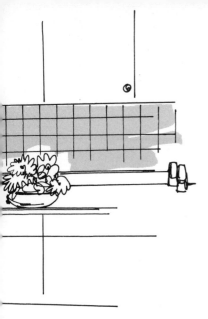

THE MILD DIABETIC

Often the term "mild" diabetes, is interpreted by the patient to mean, a mild treatment.

Diabetics, other than the mild type, have specific symptoms which demand control, and the control itself often presents problems to which the doctor and patient, must give their all.

When the doctor applies the term "mild," it usually means that control is relatively easy, and foods and insulin are easily digested and absorbed. When this occurs, the diabetic is indeed fortunate.

Because the rise in sugar in the "mild" diabetic, may not be as severe, an oral compound may be adequate for his control. If insulin is necessary, then probably a small quantity, once a day, may suffice. As a rule, this patient rarely experiences an insulin reaction.

Every diabetic would like to be a "mild" one. There are, however, a few things for the mild diabetic to think about.

We find so often in life, that those things which glitter, are not always gold. It is possible for the "mild" diabetic to feel so free of problems and complications, that he minimizes the need for control and slips into a few loose habits.

Remember, diabetes is subtle and silent. While the patient may be enjoying a less restricted life, his diabetes may be marching on.

The term "mild" as used by the doctor is correct, but may be misinterpreted by the patient. Because the diabetic does not FEEL the need for a rigid control, he is lulled into a laxity which may in time, reveal that the "napping hare" has lost the race.

Sometime ago, a woman visited her doctor, and was told she was running sugar, but by keeping to a strict diet, she could control the situation and would not have to take insulin.

The doctor explained, "You have a 'mild' case of diabetes and it is up to you to control it, with the food you eat." The doctor was right, but the woman returned home in a gay spirit. "Just a little sugar," she glibly reported. "The doctor says the case is very mild, so there is nothing to worry about." She, like many "mild" diabetics, minimized the severity of her case.

One doctor put it this way. "A person either has diabetes or he does not. The degree of severity makes no difference in the RIGIDITY OF CONTROL, whether by insulin and diet, oral compounds and diet, or by diet alone."

Cooperation between the patient and the doctor is just as important for the "mild" diabetic as the severe one. The doctor is trying to prevent a mild case from becoming severe, and a severe case from becoming fatal. He is also trying desperately to prevent additional complications, which he knows may accompany uncontrolled diabetes, whether mild or advanced.

Since a well-controlled diabetic may develop complications, think how easy a mild diabetic can develop them, if his control is lax.

In fact, doctors tell us, that some complications are apt to be more prevalent in the "mild" cases, than in the advanced. Severe diabetics are "forced" into adequate control; "mild" diabetics would do well to do likewise!

The mother of a friend of Jolene's, was not feeling well. Her doctor reported that her discomfort was caused by sugar in the urine. She was put on a strict diet and was able to control the sugar. With this control, she received relief from her problem.

With the discomfort gone, she began to slip back into her old eating habits, and soon the same trouble returned. Because she had neglected her diet, she was ashamed to return to the same doctor, so she sought out another. The new doctor diagnosed her case the same way and put her on the same strict diet.

Again, by adhering to the diet, her trouble disappeared, and for several months she was weaving back and forth between sugar, trouble and diet. Jolene asked one day, "Well, how is the diet coming?"

"Oh, fine," she responded. "You know, I have a very mild case of diabetes. If I have trouble I just go on the diet and everything clears up."

When Jolene suggested that she purchase her own testing equipment, and make at least two tests a day, she said, "Well, my doctor gave me a list of things like that to buy, but I lost the list and now I'm afraid to ask him for another."

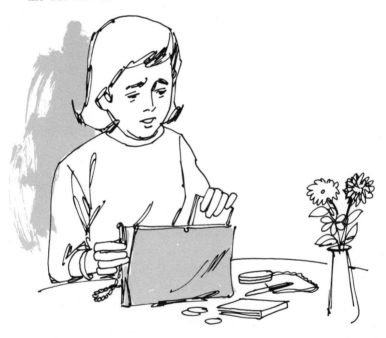

She was playing with fire, that was sure. She had not stopped to consider that the diabetes was probably becoming worse, and damage to many parts of her body was taking place.

If we were to exchange selfishness and self-will, for cooperation with the doctor, and would add to this a complete diabetic education it would pay high dividends for the rest of our lives.

A middle-aged man once said, "I have had diabetes and taken insulin for 25 years, but have never known what an insulin reaction is!"

How lucky can one man be? For a great many diabetics, this is unheard of, but true! His case is "mild," and because he maintained his daily control, he earned his reward!

The "mild" diabetic needs to remember that although the severity of the diabetes may not increase, the need for adequate control is continuous.

"Mild Diabetes" Does Not Mean "Mild Treatment,"
But Daily Adherence to the Rules as Prescribed
by the Doctor!

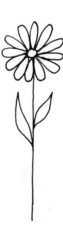

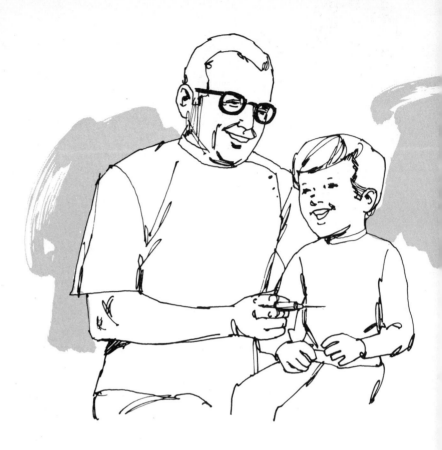

I took young Jack upon my knee,
He was so small, just over three.

I showed him how to hold the "gun"
How he might take his insulin.

Now I'm proud of that young elf,
For he wants to take it, by himself.

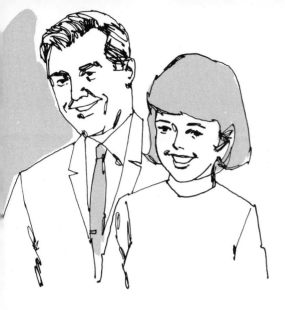

THE CHILD DIABETIC

Some children are born with diabetes, while others develop it, in their first tender years of life.

When a child has diabetes it means the pancreas is not functioning at all. Without insulin, his illness is fatal. With adequate control, the child can enjoy a useful and normal life.

We often hear the remark, "Isn't it too bad, when children develop diabetes!" Yes, it is too bad when children are handicapped with any illness, but when we compare children's diseases, there are many that are more undesirable than diabetes.

So don't feel discouraged if your child has diabetes. It just means, that for the time being, you must surmount obstacles which otherwise would not have been included in your role as parent.

You must lead the child into a happy attitude, towards his condition. Teach him the spirit of cooperation, and from the very beginning, train him to take his own injections. You will be glad you did. Measuring the quantity can be taught later.

As soon as he is old enough, teach him to make and analyze the urine tests. As soon as he can write, train him to keep his daily record.

One woman was heard to say, "My nephew has had diabetes ever since he was five years old. He is eighteen now. I have always prepared his food, given him his injections, in fact, I have never permitted him to even watch, while I administer them. This has tied me down so much that I have never been able to marry." She looked as though at any moment she expected a halo to nestle on her head.

This woman didn't realize that what she thought was a great kindness to the nephew, was only handicapping the boy. For years he had been deprived of his independence and the training which is imperative to diabetic living. In addition, he probably developed an inferiority complex.

Try to train the child to place his interest in hobbies and activities which remove his thoughts from himself, and at the same time, instill into his mind the importance of routine diabetic living. Then, you will be helping him.

Fear must not be in the child's mind, therefore it must not be in yours. The diabetic child must be made to feel that his living is no different from that of any other child, and "your happy approach" to all circumstances will create confidence in himself and you.

Make the child's meals attractive. The planning of the meal is usually done by the mother and she must be very wise and thoughtful. Here are a few suggestions.

Younger children may be fed before the rest of the family. It doesn't help the situation to have the child see his family partake of lemon meringue pie and he be given an apple or orange.

True, the day will come, when he will actually prefer the fruit, but he hasn't learned that yet. So be thoughtful, "avoiding" disappointments is easier than "explaining" them.

Use colorful dishes, changing the color and size of the dishes with each meal. Fiesta ware is good for this purpose and is not expensive.

His attention will be drawn to the dishes and he will not be as apt to notice the similarity, nor the quantity, of his foods. If the dish is too large, the serving may appear too small. This doesn't go over very well either.

Use a glass with painted palm trees, for orange or grapefruit juice. Again, do not have a large size glass for a small amount of juice. Add to the attraction by telling him the story of where these fruits are grown.

Doctors tell us that diabetic children are often unusually bright, so don't underestimate your child's mental capacity.

The training of the diabetic child should be carried on gradually, without making it a big issue. For instance, when teaching him about food, let him choose the food he wants. Teach him to measure his milk and bread, and let him select his own piece of meat. As soon as he can read, teach him the value of exchange lists. Try to make a game out of teaching the child important facts about food values.

In later years, as a college student, business executive, school teacher, accountant, or whatever place he may fill in life, he will be able to read a menu and interpret his needs correctly as he moves through a cafeteria line. His intelligent selection of food will be an asset all his life.

Mothers and fathers of these grown children, should feel well repaid for the conscientious training they have given them through childhood.

Jolene Jordan is grateful for her early training in food values which came through Dr. Elliott P. Joslin's "Diabetic Manual." She never ceased to thank him for making it possible to understand foods and convert them into a well balanced diet.

ONLY THE MOTHER KNOWS

DO NOT PERMIT well meaning friends and neighbors to feed your diabetic child. One woman said, "Mrs. Johnson always wants to feed Jimmy. She knows he has diabetes, but doesn't seem to understand the importance of diet control. I should ask her not to feed Jimmy, but I don't want to hurt her feelings." Generally speaking, it is a wise policy not to feed any child at any time, unless requested by the mother.

There is no mother in all the world, who has a greater right, than the mother of a diabetic child, to go directly to a Mrs. Johnson, diplomatically, yet emphatically to state that Jimmy is not to be fed one mouthful of food away from home. Mrs. Johnson may even say, "Oh, don't give it a second thought, it wasn't cookies. It was only an apple."

It is difficult to make someone like this understand that an apple contains sugar, and that your Jimmy does not have sufficient insulin to cover this extra food.

Repeated instances like this could mean that Jimmy's very life is at stake. There is also the risk of breaking down the diabetic training the parents have been building, hour-by-hour. If everyone could understand this, it would make the diabetic life easier for the children.

Adult diabetics have been warned to give careful attention to their feet, because of decreased circulation. This fact is important to the child also. Don't permit the diabetic child to "outgrow" his shoes, or to wear shoes that rub blisters on his feet, or are too long or too short for him.

It is important that he be taken to a good podiatrist, to have his feet analyzed for the proper size and type of shoe, best suited to him. Next, take him to a reputable shop for a perfect fit. The few extra dollars required to care for his feet, should never be considered a barrier. Always remember the grim fact that you can never buy a new foot.

Do not make diabetes the main subject of conversation in the home. Everyone tires of it. The child diabetic may develop a self-conscious approach to his condition, which could affect his ability to take his place in society. The gradual approach of playing it cool, is still the best and only way.

If the child is quite young, he may enjoy these rhymes:

I'm always thankful when I eat,
Because my food is hard to beat.
I like my eggs and milk and toast,
In fact, I like each one the most.

My butter is so yellow,
Just like the shining sun.
I'll eat it all, then I can play
And have a lot of fun.

I only eat what mother makes,
She cooks just what is best.
For then I feel so very good,
Crammed full of zip and zest.

My mother always lets me take
Some candy-mints with me,
And if I feel I'm getting weak,
I eat—say, two or three.

I do each day what mother says,
Stay closely by her side.
I know when Daddy comes at night
He'll hug me tight, with pride.

The child might enjoy this rhyme at the time of taking his insulin injection.

My mother called, I must go in,
It's time to take my insulin.
I hold the "thing-a-ma-jig" just so,
It's like a little gun, you know.
My Daddy says I'll grow to be
A man as big and tall as he.

For the little girl, the last two lines may read:

My Daddy says I'll grow to be
Just like my Mom, as fine as she.

When you tuck the child in bed at night, it might be well to suggest, he include in his bedtime prayer, thankfulness for life and happiness, his doctor, the nurse in the doctor's office, good food, his father and mother who take such good care of him, and an earnest request to be helpful to his friends.

At best, child rearing calls upon parents to be many things, but to rear a diabetic child calls for an even greater love and understanding than is usually demanded.

Happiness in the home is a must, for diabetics can only be happy and grow, in happy surroundings.

Here's a Salute to the Parents Who Have
Met This Challenge, and Won!

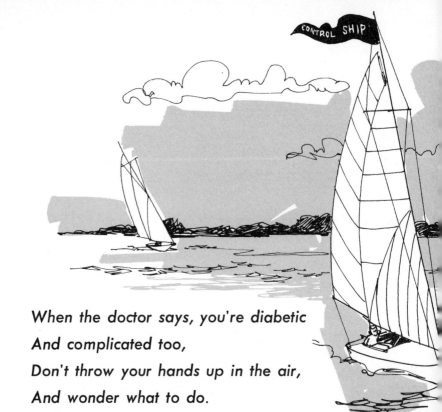

When the doctor says, you're diabetic
And complicated too,
Don't throw your hands up in the air,
And wonder what to do.

From day to day, just seek to find
Success in good control.
Don't give up the ship of health,
Before you reach your goal.

Stay calm, and try to set your sail,
For a sailor you must be.
Control your ship, so you can sail
That diabetic sea!

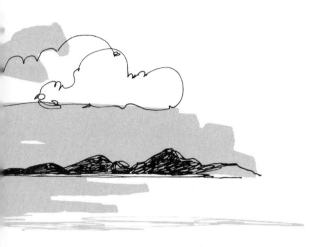

THE COMPLICATED DIABETIC

Ordinarily, the term "complicated" refers to diabetics who have developed hardening of the arteries, kidney trouble, heart trouble, gangrene, changes in the eyes, or any of the serious complications resulting from uncontrolled sugar, or diabetes of long duration. The brittle, hard to control, and as a result, complicated diabetic, is included in this category.

Controlling the sugar of a complicated diabetic is like trying to pick up quicksilver. So far, the diabetic's questions have been "what" and "when," but the complicated diabetic must also ask "why," "which" and "what for," because he REALLY has a panther in his pocket.

He has found that the schedule of a carefully weighed or measured diet and a uniform amount of insulin, which worked well for three or four days, has suddenly crumbled. The tests may have changed to a four-plus, indicating a rise in the blood sugar level, which even additional amounts of insulin have failed to control.

Then again, after three or four days of running the four-plus, the tests may suddenly show a turn into the opposite direction. They may run from a sugar-freeness that goes beyond the "life-saver mint" stage for control, to repeated antidotes of orange juice (with sugar added), or a candy bar.

This sugar-free condition may continue for several days, and then once more, sugar may show up in the tests.

These erratic and unpredictable changes in the blood sugar level, pave the way to a more rapid hardening of the arteries, which precipitate neuritis, blindness, gangrene and many other unwanted complications of diabetes.

The resolvement of this diabetic problem, involves amount of insulin, food, timing, exercise, and anything else that may enter the area of control. The problems of the complicated diabetic can and must be conquered.

No one knows why some cases of diabetes are so difficult to control. Only the patient, close family members, and the experienced doctor, understand the complete problem.

With either of the two extremes just mentioned, a few or all of the following symptoms may appear: dizziness, confusion, problems in balance, disturbance in vision, feeling of nausea, aches through the body, and a general feeling of "I just want to lie down."

Be sure to talk these problems over with your doctor. He has knowledge and wide experience to draw from, and can make many suggestions towards a solution.

It has been discovered that the blood sugar and urine sugar of a complicated diabetic do not always stay together. Normally, when the blood sugar goes up, the urine sugar goes up with it. But, complications come when the blood sugar goes up or down and the urine does not reflect this change.

The only test available to the diabetic at home is the urine test, and when he tries to suit control to the test results, he runs into trouble. We are told, some day it may be possible for the diabetic to determine his blood sugar with a simple test at home.

In the meantime, if a complicated diabetic is observed eating between meals, don't bombard him with questions. Trust him, he knows his needs.

Someone may try to tell you that you make errors in drawing the insulin into the syringe or in the dosage.

It is difficult for the diabetic to listen to such accusations. Granting the fact that making a mistake in the amount of insulin is always possible, there is another fact just as true. All diabetics, and especially the complicated ones, check and recheck each amount, before injection, because they are fully aware of the results, should there be a mistake.

There are those, who in an attempt to sound knowledgeable, tell you, it is impossible to get an accurate and uniform amount of insulin each time, because a certain percentage of the insulin may cling to the barrel of the syringe.

This is another irresponsible statement. If it is said to you, don't let it throw you. This is a "uniform condition" that exists with every shot of insulin. The calibration on the syringe is the diabetic's confidence. Make sure the syringe is dry inside, draw the amount prescribed, check it, and "thank Heaven" you have it to take.

When insulin was first used by diabetics in the home, a specific schedule was given him to follow, a weighed (gram) diet, a specific amount of insulin at a certain time, and moderate exercise. He was expected to continue on this schedule every day, and was led to believe his success was assured. However, in the years of experience that followed, the thinking of the medical world and the diabetic world has enlarged to include these facts:

Every diabetic is different.

Some types of insulin are not suitable for some diabetics.

That other illnesses, major or minor, affect control.

Education of the patient, his ability to apply it, are vital.

Control is easier when the weight of the diabetic is normal.

That chemical changes in the body, may change control.

That exercise plays a major role.

That fatigue adds a strain on control.

That certain drugs affect control.

That the diabetic's emotions affect control and vice versa.

That attitude, cooperativeness, cheerfulness, are important.

That changes in seasons affect control.

That certain areas of the country, especially the warm south, are more conducive to good control.

When science indicated that these outside factors influenced the control of diabetes, in addition to the suspected failure of the patient, then the control of diabetes took another step forward.

Several years ago, a diabetic sought help at a source, quite a distance from home. After the usual days of tests and observations, he was sent home with a prescribed diet, amount of insulin, and instructions to lose 25 pounds.

Over a period of two years, the 25 pounds were lost, eight changes of seasons were hurdled, two severe colds combated and overcome. The weight loss, the seasons, the colds—combined with a seriously complicated control, demanded many changes in the schedule suggested two years before.

Upon his return to the source of help, he heard the complaint that this was not the program prescribed two years ago. Remembering some of the deep valleys encountered, he listened and could only breathe a prayer of thanksgiving that life still flowed in his veins.

Today, this lack of understanding of the problems of complicated diabetes has changed, and each diabetic is treated individually.

In this area, an understanding spouse or parent, can be of great help to the complicated diabetic.

Jolene can recall that while visiting a clinic several years ago, her husband decided unexpectedly to visit her for the weekend. He placed several oranges in his brief-case before leaving home, "just in case."

When he arrived and knocked on her door, there was no answer. Repeated knockings brought no results. Finally the door was forced open and he found her unconscious from too low a blood sugar. The husband's oranges worked well, and Jolene has always been thankful for the unexpected visit of a thoughtful husband.

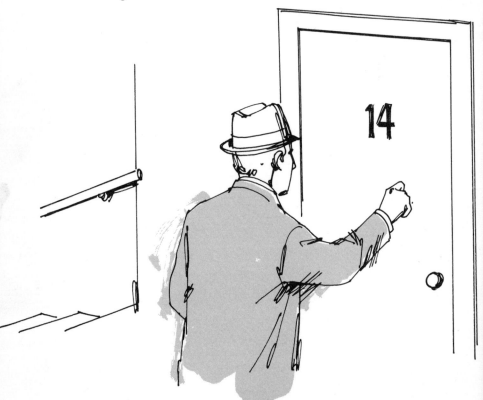

The everyday life of a complicated diabetic is more restricted since the control is tighter. But when he becomes adjusted to his schedule, he is free to enter into every phase of normal living.

Many times, his restrictions become an asset, for he learns many lessons, which others fail to learn.

It also seems, because of the strict control, into which he is forced, certain areas of his body are better preserved. Rapid deterioration which many diabetics, living in loose control experience, does not occur.

Every cloud **DOES** have a silver lining, and the silver lining for the complicated diabetic is insulin. Without it, daisies would soon grow above him, and those daisies would never tell of the life he might have enjoyed with his loved ones.

It Doesn't REALLY Hurt!

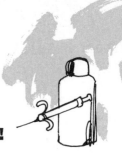

The doctor is speaking with ominous sound,
My heart keeps rolling, around and around.

"High sugar," he says.—"Start treatment today."
Treatment means insulin—I cannot obey!

High sugar, I thought, was Aunt Helen's trouble.
"High sugar," I murmur, my mind's in a muddle.

Take insulin? With a needle? I shiver and shudder.
"I'll never do that!" And on this, I don't stutter.

The doctor looks stern, with his eyes of cold steel.
"You'll do it TODAY—before your next meal."

I break in a sweat, and withdraw in a huddle.
By noon I'm a wreck, and STILL in a muddle.

Just then he returns with determined set face,
And looks like the bull, on Uncle Jack's place.

I want to run fast, never see him again,
Because he just looks, like the coldest of men.

Surely and quickly, this man of cold steel,
Gets ready to show me, that "Insulin Deal."

He puts the syringe in my cold, clammy fist,
Calmly guiding my hand, but firm, from the wrist!

—"I did it!—'T'was easy!" I cry with high glee,
The doctor's steel eyes—now blue, look at me.

Why, he was handsome and gentle, the best doctor yet!
High sugar?—Take insulin?—Bring it on!—I'm all set!

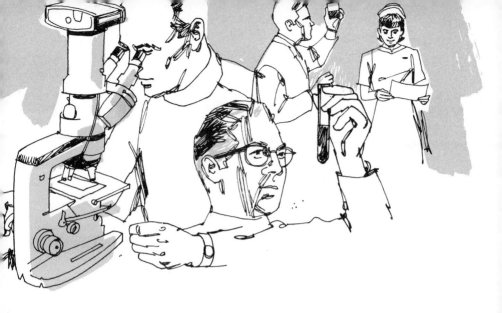

INSULIN—The Pancreas In A Bottle

About 1915, when Jolene's brother was a small boy, he exhibited symptoms of diabetes, and well does she recall her grandmother, with solemn eyes, saying to her mother, "Has it ever occurred to you, he may have diabetes?" Jolene's mother nodded her head and looking into the distance, said, "Yes, it would be a terrible thing." All day, gloom sat in the home, and a trip to the doctor the following day resulted in the assurance he did NOT have diabetes.

The memory of that day returned to Jolene, several years later, in 1932, when an exhausting weakness and overpowering thirst drove her to the doctor, and she heard him say, "You have diabetes."

But in those intervening years, between her brother's reprieve and her own apprehension, two doctors, Frederick Grant Banting and Charles Herbert Best, and their research staff, had merged their dreams with labor, and gave the world the priceless gift of insulin. This discovery changed a disease of dread and death, into a life of usefulness and happiness.

A BIT OF HISTORY

Much research had been done by many scientists prior to the time of Dr. Banting and Dr. Best, but none was successful in its application to the human body. After many heart-breaking failures, in 1921 these two scientists experienced their first glimmer of hope.

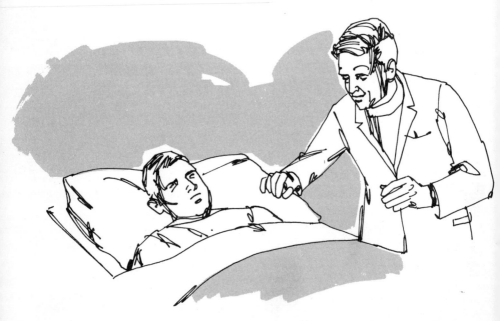

In 1922, Dr. Banting injected the first human being with insulin, Joe Gilchrist, one of his childhood friends. Joe Gilchrist was a severe diabetic and barely survived on a scant diet, he was extremely emaciated at the time of the first insulin injection on February 11, 1922.

What a thrill it must have been to the patient, to feel strength enter his body once more, and what a thrill for Dr. Banting and Dr. Best and their associates!

Next, came the period of refining the impure product, which they were able to do, after many successes and many failures. Because of the risk of infection at the injection site, it was necessary for the patient to live in the hospital until 1928. From then on, the diabetic was allowed to live at home and administer his own insulin.

Diabetics throughout the world, heard of the new medicine and the demand was staggering. New sources had to be found, and it was at this time the discovery was made, that insulin could be taken from the pancreas of cattle and pork.

Research continued until there were two types of insulin, then three, and in 1937 the first "long lasting" insulin was discovered. This enabled many diabetics to reduce their three and four daily shots of insulin, to one.

Because this still did not meet the needs of all diabetics, it was found that the "short" and "long" lasting insulins could be combined, thereby, with one shot, supply immediate as well as later coverage of the rising blood sugar.

The development had come a long, long way. Many lives were snatched from death, and turned into rich and rewarding living, with normal desires and normal fulfillment. Figuratively speaking, diabetics and their loved ones, danced in the street, and sang.

To ease the living still further, for some diabetics, in 1957, an oral compound to control the blood sugar, was introduced. At first, there was some resistance, but it was found that many adult diabetics could use it quite successfully, and in recent years additional oral controls have been placed on the market. The diabetics who find them adequate, are jubilant, and it is hoped that some day the control for all diabetics will be as simple.

There is great anticipation at present, that before too many years have passed, pancreas transplants will be used to cure diabetes. Should this hope become fact, it would be a great day for the diabetic. But until that day comes, we have much living to do, and every diabetic is eager to do his part, in up-holding the standards of diabetic living, that he may be worthy of whatever the future holds.

Research continues on the cause of and cure for diabetes. It is one of the most baffling mysteries scientists have faced.

In the meantime, let us consider some of the ways in which diabetics can live better each day with insulin.

When a diabetic is first told he must take insulin, and that the only way of administering it, is by hypodermic injection, no one can deny that his first reaction is one of stunned unbelief.

But skilled and kind doctors, understand this very important and necessary "first" lesson. They hold the key to giving the diabetic the proper introduction and attitude towards what at first, seems horrifying and impossible to do.

If any diabetic, prior to his onset of diabetes, were asked if
he could give himself an injection of insulin, he would probably
have said something like, "Count me out, I could NEVER
do it."

But each diabetic knows when the time comes, he must be
strong and brave. In his eagerness to retain his independence
and experience the control he needs, he discovers that self-
administration is the ONLY way to maintain happy diabetic
living.

There may be two circumstances when the injection should
be given by someone else.

1. In case of an emergency, or where the eyesight is inade-
quate, there should always be someone in the home, trained
to measure the insulin into the syringe and injecting it. This
should be the only reason, a diabetic may call on a family
member.

2. When the diabetic is a patient in the hospital, it is a welcome relief to have the nurse inject the insulin. Apart from the
fact it gives added rest and relaxation to the patient, the injection site can be changed. The diabetic, as a rule, uses the thigh
for the injection, but the nurse can inject it into the upper arm.

Changing the place of injection is extremely important. If
insulin is injected into the same area each time, soon a hard
mass forms and eventually may have to be removed, surgically.

A nurse reminded Jolene of this fact, saying, "Be sure to
keep moving the site of injection. I have a nurse friend who is

diabetic, and recently she had to come to the hospital and have a hard mass of tissue removed from each leg where she continuously injected the insulin." She continued with, "I just can't get over it! That a nurse who has been taught so differently, could do something like that!"

Jolene, like all insulin-taking diabetics, understood what had been the diabetic nurse's problem. There is an area at the top front of each thigh where the needle can be slipped in very easily, almost without feeling. It is a temptation to use this area each time. But this is where the trouble begins.

That's why doctors remind us many times—

▶ KEEP MOVING THE SITE OF INJECTION,
IT IS IMPORTANT!

If the diabetic is a child, choosing a new spot for injection can become a game. The child will not think about the injection as much as the choice, and before you know it, the injection is done.

It is suggested, when holding the syringe in your hands prior to injection, while pushing the plunger up and down to remove moisture inside the barrel, that you hold the top of the needle with the left hand, as the up and down pressure sometimes forces the needle from the syringe. When this happens, the point is blunted and the needle dulled. This causes a delay by having to sterilize a NEW needle. Here, disposable needles have an advantage.

Getting the correct amount of insulin is so important, that a double check is justified. If you take more than one kind, check each bottle carefully, BEFORE you draw it from the bottle, and AFTERWARD. Don't permit your thoughts to wander, or let some distraction cause you to question what you actually drew into the syringe. BE SURE YOU ARE SURE!

If a specified time for taking insulin is prescribed by your doctor, be sure to stick to this schedule, and let nothing interfere.

Don't change the amount of insulin without checking with your doctor. Or, if he permits you to make these adjustments when necessary, be sure the record you give him on your next visit, reflects the amount of insulin taken, and the test results.

If the doctor has given you this permission, it is well to develop a pattern that works uniformly, rather than changing the amount frequently. Doctors usually discourage the diabetic from changing the amount frequently.

Jolene often recalls Dr. Joslin's words, in part, that there is no one who regrets a transgression of the rules, for diabetic living, more than the diabetic himself. When he does try to experiment with what might appear to be a more pleasurable diet or an improved insulin dosage, or way of life, it doesn't take him long to get back into the harness. Believe me, a repentant diabetic has a memory like an elephant.

Diabetic doctors often tell us that anything involved in the treatment of the diabetic should not be "too little" or "too much." In other words, play it cool. Too tight or compulsive treatment is no better than too loose a control.

One woman said her husband ate everything he wanted and then took enough insulin to cover. Many doctors agree, this is not good control, and that this man is poorly adjusted and some day will pay a heavy price with many body failures which could have been avoided with a controlled diet and stabilized amount of insulin. Insulin was given to use, not abuse.

Jolene Jordan discovered that when her weight was a couple of pounds under normal, and she ate minimum but adequate food, took minimum but adequate insulin, and included moderate exercise, she felt better.

The body functions best, with the correct amount of insulin and food.

Insulin reactions are kept to a minimum with a well regulated schedule.

Keep the insulin equipment in the most convenient place you can find, and keep the syringe and needle sterilized at all times.

Be sure to keep extra needles and syringes on hand, and know where they are.

Disposable syringes have become quite popular because of convenience.

Understanding the syringe is a must, and there are many kinds on the market.

One day, Jolene was in a Medical Supply House, when a man approached her, took a syringe from his vest pocket, and said, "I was just released from the hospital this morning and have never taken insulin before. They gave me this syringe and told me how to use it, but I just can't remember what they said. Would you look at it and explain to me how it works?"

Jolene looked at it, and although she was acquainted with two or three types, had never seen anything like this one before. She suggested he call his doctor, and get instructions from him only. A new diabetic with a syringe in his hands, he doesn't understand, is a pathetic sight.

Your doctor will advise and teach you about the syringe best suited to your needs.

KEEP EXTRA INSULIN ON HAND

NEVER let your supply of insulin run down to the last bottle. This may be the time an accident may occur, and may also be the time, the store is closed.

Jolene recalls the emergency message that went out over the radio in Chicago the morning of the Great Snow in January 1967. A woman called the station to say, her father had taken the last of his insulin supply, the day before, and had planned to go to the drug store that morning.

But, of course, during the night the snow fell, doors of homes could not be opened, the sidewalks could not be found, streets were impassible, owners of stores could not reach them, and there sat a diabetic who had failed to assume his responsibility of seeing to it, that there was an extra bottle of insulin on hand. (In fact, at that moment, he should have had two extra bottles, in case of breakdown.) Diabetes does not wait.

The druggist was forced to make an almost impossible trip to the store, digging his way as he went. A special messenger had to be called and sent to the diabetic's home with the insulin, digging his way also as he went. Someone at home had to rush the almost unbelievable job of scooping out the entrance to the home. What a fiasco, instead of adequate preparation!

She also remembers a diabetic woman, who visited a nearby city where stores closed promptly at 9 PM and opened at 9 AM. She stayed in a hotel, became ill during the night, and decided she needed more insulin. She had one bottle with her, which in her ill condition, dropped to the floor while trying to extract the insulin. The hotel management had to be aroused, the druggist (as in the story just related) was aroused and made his trips, including delivery to the hotel.

An added concern might have been—WHAT IF THE DRUGGIST HAD NOT HAD IN STOCK, THE SPECIFIC INSULIN NEEDED?

These happenings should never occur. Diabetics must think ahead and be prepared for any emergency. This is one of the many MUSTS.

Another kind of insulin emergency befell a small diabetic child in Wyoming. Her father traveled from their ranch to a nearby city for insulin. He spent a couple of days in a bar, and after having much too much to drink, took a bottle of insulin from his pocket, waved it in the air, and shouted through thick lips, "Do you see this? It is for my little girl at home. She needs it."

When he arrived at home the following day, the little girl didn't need it anymore.

The need for insulin is instant and delay of control can bring only one result.

To Sum up:

1. ALWAYS HAVE AN EXTRA BOTTLE OF INSULIN ON HAND.

2. ALWAYS CARRY INSULIN, SYRINGE AND NEEDLES WITH YOU—WHEREVER YOU GO!

When a diabetic is scheduled to go to the doctor for a blood sugar, the patient must not change his insulin or food intake in any way, in an effort to secure better test results. When a true test is not obtained, the real condition will not be known. Also, it could take a couple of days to get the unruly blood sugar back on schedule. This is NOT good diabetic living.

Do not take more insulin than you need, expecting to eat extra food. This irregularity can also throw the control off for several days.

Much attention has been given recently to what is called "loose control." Some authorities have felt, that a rigid control has its handicaps, and that a loose control, with a certain amount of insulin and food, chosen at the discretion of the diabetic, may be helpful.

Emotionally, this may have an advantage, but many diabetics with experience, are of the opinion, that a set amount of insulin and food, carefully selected by the doctor, is by far the better way.

All diabetics know only too well, how quickly a half-cup can look too small, and how easy it is for a piece of meat to grow from average size to a large size. With no restraint, and with freedom of choice, it would be very easy for a diabetic to fall into difficulty.

The term "loose" does not help at all, for it indicates a freedom which in reality does not exist.

One morning when Jolene arrived at her office, she was met by a sad faced young woman, who was usually quite gay.

"Well, good morning," Jolene greeted her.

Without responding, the young woman slipped her arm around Jolene and said, "I've just been told you are a diabetic."

"Yes, I am," confirmed Jolene.

The sympathy of her co-worker increased. "I'm so sorry to hear it. We like you so much here. How long does the doctor give you?"

Jolene was stunned, however, she was sympathetic with her friend, because she realized that the horrible stories of a diabetic's existence were still being told, even in this new and enlightened age.

Jolene consoled her friend, "That isn't true anymore. Insulin has been given the diabetic to help his failing pancreas, and by living discreetly, he can live a full and normal life every day, in every way."

"I didn't know," smiled the friend. "Medicine is wonderful!"

The older and the more experienced a diabetic becomes, the greater is his appreciation for what insulin has meant to the world.

INSULIN IS THE LIFE-LINE OF THE DIABETIC!

Thank you again, Dr. Banting and Dr. Best.

INSULIN SHOCK (Reactions)

When the blood sugar drops too low, the resulting experience is called an insulin shock, or insulin reaction. It is well named. The drop may have been caused by taking too much insulin, an omission of some food in the diet, a delayed meal, or may be some excessive exercise. Also, some prescribed medicines have been known to lower the blood sugar. Your doctor will know which may be true in your case.

Every diabetic is warned by his doctor, to avoid insulin reactions.

There are several stages of insulin shock. They range all the way from a dull headache to unconsciousness.

SYMPTOMS OF INSULIN SHOCK: Weakness, excessive perspiration, tingling tongue, confusion, faintness, trembling, blurring of vision, laughing or crying without cause, talking thickly, staggering drunkenly, yes, the patient may even become unconscious, if help is not immediate.

ANTIDOTES FOR INSULIN SHOCK: If the reaction occurs at home, the best antidote is orange juice. If the reaction is severe, add two teaspoons of sugar.

If away from home, and orange juice IS available, use it. If it is not, then sugared water, tea, coffee, or sugared soft drinks will work well. As diabetics are expected to carry lumps of sugar or candy with them at all times, and if conscious, they can help themselves to recover. If someone is aiding the patient, he can place the sugar under his tongue. Many consider this to be the safest antidote, when the patient is unconscious and unable to swallow.

If the diabetic is unconscious, and it is unknown whether he is in insulin shock or diabetic coma, he should be rushed to the nearest hospital. They will know how to diagnose the problem and administer the correct antidote. The patient's doctor will be called by the hospital.

After a diabetic has had one or two experiences with insulin shock, he learns to recognize the first wave of weakness, and intercept the progress with a small amount of orange juice or one or two candy mints, which often will hold a mild reaction in abeyance until mealtime.

Since every diabetic is different, the doctor will prescribe the amount and type of insulin, and the amount of food, best suited to his needs. When the diabetic indulges in a long walk, cleans the house, mows the lawn, plays a round of golf, or participates in any form of excessive exercise, the doctor may advise eating something prior to the exercise or reducing the amount of insulin.

Of course, this does not mean a five-course dinner, but rather an orange or a couple of life-saver mints. It is also suggested that the diabetic place a package of mints in his pocket, if the exercise is being taken, outside of the home.

When the diabetic needs sugar to counteract an insulin reaction, he is usually not able, emotionally, to discuss why he must eat the candy at that moment.

Give him the opportunity to eat it. It is impossible for him to chew, swallow, and carry on a conversation. His emotional system cannot tolerate it. He needs food more than anything else at that moment, and by leaving him alone, you are doing him the greatest kindness.

DO NOT SEEK TO ENGAGE A DIABETIC IN CONVER-
SATION WHEN YOU SEE HIM EATING CANDY. THIS
IS HELPFUL ADVICE!

Don't worry about the diabetic doing some cheating. He
knows better than anyone else that cheating makes him the
loser. He knows only too well the feeling of a "cottony" dry
mouth, a weak body, a severe headache, and a nauseated stomach. He wants to avoid these, a thousand times more than anyone else could ever know. Keep trusting him, he will be a
much happier and better controlled diabetic, and yes, the whole
family will be happier too.

Everyone needs to understand the need for antidotes for diabetic control. Every diabetic who has had to resort to sugar,
has heard someone say, "A diabetic eating candy? Well, no
wonder he was in the hospital last winter, and so sick too!"

The critic doesn't understand the value of this piece of candy.
It prevented a much more serious complication, perhaps helped
to save the diabetic's life.

A young woman, after discovering that Jolene was diabetic,
said, "I had an uncle who had diabetes. And you know, no
matter how much we talked to him, he always carried a candy
bar in his pocket." Opening her eyes wide and looking almost
threateningly at Jolene, said, "And he died!"

Jolene smiled inwardly and at the same time felt concern
for the lack of diabetic education among the public in general. How could Jolene convince this strong opinionated young
woman that no wise diabetic, who takes insulin or the oral
compounds, is ever very far away from some form of sugar?

The candy bar, the uncle carried and ate when he needed it, did not cause his death; but rather, prolonged his life. The nagging family did him much harm.

It is true, before the discovery of insulin, the only known control for diabetes was the restriction of sugar and starches in the diet, almost to the point of starvation. Many UNinformed people still carry the impression that diabetics must not include sugars or starches in their diet and control.

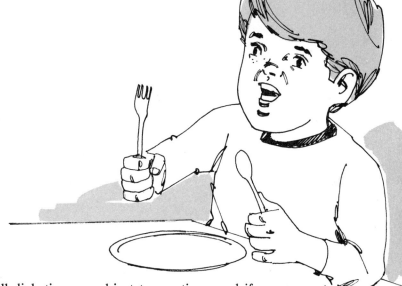

Not all diabetics are subject to reactions, and if you are not, be grateful, for there are thousands who battle this complication daily. If you are subject to reactions, keep yourself alert.

A three-year-old diabetic boy was quite brittle, but his mother reported that after he had two or three insulin reactions, he learned to recognize them and would run in from the yard, climb into his chair at the table, and call out, "Eat! Eat!"

The mother never questioned him, but gave him orange juice without delay, let him sit at the table after drinking the juice, without talking. In about five minutes he would return to the yard, with his usual vigor. A later test always proved he knew what he was doing.

A diabetic should discipline himself to speak up, the instant the first nervous tremor of an insulin reaction is felt. If the reaction is not treated promptly, the patient may go into unconsciousness.

As a rule, the experienced diabetic can keep an insulin reaction under control, but there is always the possibility that he can lapse into unconsciousness and be at the mercy of those around him.

> THEREFORE, EVERY DIABETIC SHOULD HAVE LUMPS OF SUGAR OR A CANDY BAR IN HIS POCKET OR PURSE, AT ALL TIMES, AND AN IDENTIFICATION CARD IN HIS WALLET, BEARING HIS NAME, ADDRESS, PHONE NUMBER, AND NAME OF NEAREST KIN WITH PHONE NUMBER, AND NAME OF HIS DOCTOR, ADDRESS, AND TELEPHONE NUMBER. BE SURE TO INCLUDE THE TYPE AND AMOUNT OF INSULIN, AND TIME SCHEDULE.

It has been suggested that it be mandatory for all diabetics to wear an identification wristband that opens like a watch, with the above information, and an obvious "DIABETIC" marked on it.

The American Medical Association has this to say about the important subject of proper identification for diabetics:

"There are three instances in which knowledge that a person is a diabetic might aid those assisting him, in doing the right thing.

"One of these is the hypoglycemic reaction or insulin reaction which begins with confusion simulating alcoholic intoxication and leads through convulsions to unconsciousness which could be fatal or very damaging unless immediate treatment is provided to raise the level of the blood sugar.

"Another is the exact opposite in which an individual through indiscretions or failure to take insulin develops an extremely high blood sugar frequently complicated with the presence of acetone leading to coma and requiring immediate and rather dramatic therapy.

"The third is the instance where a diabetic taking insulin suffers an injury or illness under conditions where he is not known and where he is unable to communicate the fact of his diabetes. The absence of insulin will most certainly complicate his recovery from the injury or sudden illness that he suffers.

"We believe that all diabetics should wear a durable signal device bearing the symbol of emergency medical identification and at least the word, DIABETIC.

"He should also carry an emergency medical identification card giving further details regarding his problem to further guide those who might be giving him treatment in the emergency room of a hospital."

It is suggested you consult your doctor concerning securing information from The American Medical Association of Chicago, on the signal devices and identification cards referred to.

Because of the hazards of insulin reactions and coma, doctors are beginning to believe that a middle of the road approach to controlling diabetes, is better than leaning too far to the left or to the right.

As you make your tests, remember, a test showing a trace, or even a one, may be better than a continuous zero, but that a two is quite questionable, and a three or four should be definitely avoided.

Someone has said, "When we begin pushing the human body, it has a way of pushing back." This holds true when we take in our hands the responsibility of hand-operating an unknown quantity like the pancreas, which was placed within the body for a normal specific function. The wisdom of our Creator must somehow be understood by the limited wisdom of man.

The diabetic must be relaxed and calm, planning and plotting each step of diabetic control. If he uses caution, he will not be in need of emergency treatment.

Control is not always easy, but every diabetic has been given the proper tools, and thousands upon thousands are proving every day—IT CAN BE DONE!

DIABETIC COMA

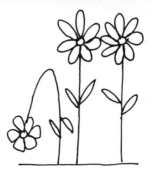

Coma could be called a "last ditch stand" as the diabetic feels backed against the wall. Some recover, others do not. Until insulin was discovered, coma accounted for over 50 percent of the diabetic deaths.

The onset of coma is slow, and during that time the patient is extremely weak and weary. He develops a dull headache which is accompanied by an insatiable thirst. It may take several weeks to reach the last stage of unconsciousness. The only remedy is insulin.

The victim may NOT KNOW he is diabetic, or may know he IS diabetic but does not recognize coma symptoms. He may not realize that diabetes must be controlled, and may be hoping it is just "something that will go away" and neglect to consult his doctor. He does not realize the panther in his pocket is ready to spring for the kill.

A diabetic goes into coma when there is too much sugar in the blood and he is not using insulin. Some, who take insulin, find the sugar rises to a four-plus during the day, perhaps in the early morning hours, and at that time discover acetone in the urine. Acetone is caused when carbohydrates (sugars and starches) are not available in the breakdown of protein and fats. Insulin enables carbohydrates to perform its part in this digestive process.

A test for acetone should be made at the same time as the test for sugar. Both tests are simple and fast. *(See "1-2-3-4 Testing Lane")*

The combination of acetone and four-plus in the urine is extremely undesirable, and may be the forerunner of coma, if allowed to continue. When acetone and high sugar coincide, extensive damage and deterioration may occur. This condition should be avoided as you would a cobra.

Acetone leads to acidosis, acidosis to coma, coma to—death.

When this condition exists, be SURE to contact your doctor and whatever adjustment is necessary in food and insulin, he will make.

A patient in the hospital said to her roommate, "You know, I have been a diabetic 26 years and have never understood about acetone."

The roommate replied, "Oh, acetone is nothing to worry about. I have heard of people who are not diabetic, and have acetone. So don't worry about that." The roommate didn't realize she was giving erroneous information, and lulling the diabetic into a false sense of security.

Some diabetics have observed acetone at the same time as sugar-freeness. This may mean they are not getting enough food to meet the amount of insulin taken, or the ratio of carbohydrates and fat is not balanced. Only your doctor can diagnose the cause in your case. However, he depends on the patient, to detect the presence of acetone.

When acetone and coma develop, there is a "sweetish fruity" odor to the breath, resembling alcohol. Doctors and members of the family can enter a room and sense that the diabetic is in difficulty. But the inexperienced by-stander, knows only that the victim is unconscious and his breath smells of alcohol.

Several years ago a woman was found unconscious in an outside doorway by two detectives. Noting her "alcoholic" breath, they assumed she had been drinking. She was taken to the

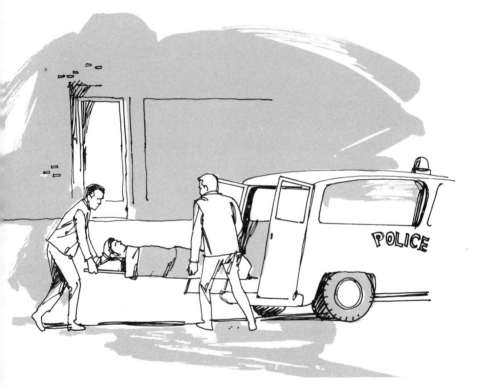

station. Although she had identification and a bottle of insulin in her purse, the diabetic was placed in a cell to "sleep it off." By morning, she was dead.

Situations of this nature are serious, and all public service personnel must be made aware of it.

When a diabetic is found unconscious, it is difficult for the uninformed onlooker to detect the cause. As previously indicated, he might be in insulin shock, which would call for sugar or orange juice as an antidote, or he might be in coma, which would call for insulin. A mistake in diagnosis and treatment, could be fatal.

All public personnel are now being trained to detect the difference between insulin shock, coma breath and alcoholic indulgence, in order that they may give immediate and proper help, to the helpless diabetic.

▶ BE SURE TO CARRY ALL THE NECESSARY INDENTIFICATION AS INDICATED IN THE PREVIOUS CHAPTER!

If uncontrolled diabetes is allowed to progress, the arteries will harden at a more rapid pace, which in turn paves the way to poor circulation, heart attacks, neuritis and blindness.

These complications may also come, at a slower pace, to the diabetic well controlled with insulin. In the light of this truth, can anyone question the importance of daily, hourly control of his diabetes? Or, the importance of early detection?

Jolene Jordan clearly remembers a coma experience, during the early days of insulin. In 1932 the symptoms were not yet generally recognized as denoting diabetes, and insulin had not yet been fully accepted as the proper control for diabetes.

In those days, ignorance of the use of insulin with diet, was rampant. Advice on all sides said, omission of sugars and starches is the only way to control diabetes. It took a trip to death's door for Jolene to prove this fallacy.

The incidence rate of coma has been reduced in the last 20 years, because doctors, nurses, associates and associations, and yes, diabetics, are bending every effort to increase the knowledge and understanding of diabetes in general, and thereby avoid the dark days of coma.

When diabetes comes to live with you, even as an unwanted guest, try to be friends, for you now have a permanent houseguest.

The severity may increase or decrease, but whichever happens, diabetes remains. If we learn to live with it from the beginning, it will ease the way, and the pitfalls will become stepping stones to a healthier, happier life on the diabetic road.

Thanks again, for insulin!

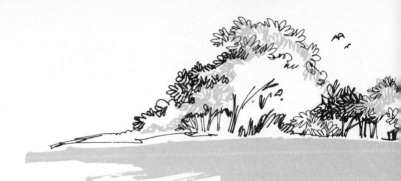

PICNICS ARE FUN

Invite ALL diabetics
To gather in the park.
And bring along: knife, fork and spoon,
For a diabetic lark.

Bring fried chicken, with potatoes,
A salad, beans and butter'd bread,
Some milk and berries, red and ripe,
For our Picnic spread.

Now it's time to eat, so gather 'round
Our meal for diabetics.
Let's ALL have fun and let us be
The PRIDE, of all our medics!

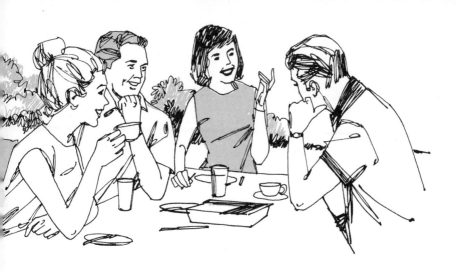

IT'S TIME TO EAT!

Eating three meals a day, one of the more pleasurable experiences of life, is enjoyed even more, when the diabetic controls his condition.

The food we eat, ranks next to insulin, in bringing about adequate control. WHAT you eat does not cause diabetes, but plays a major role in the control of it. In fact, one might say, insulin and food work hand-in-hand, ready to lead the diabetic into successful living.

The diabetic who is fortunate, to control his condition with food alone, must have just as complete a knowledge of his diet, as the one, who takes insulin or an oral compound.

Insulin and the compound have been previously prepared, and all the diabetic has to do, is take them. No worry, no fuss.

Food, is a different story.

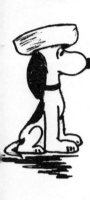

Before insulin, the diabetic's supper dish could have looked like Snoopy's—"he could have worn it on his head!"

Today, the diabetic is allowed a complete and adequate diet. Every diabetic has been given a list of foods, which make up his diet, including the proper amounts, and instructions to study and follow the list carefully.

After some study, the involved calculations may become too much for him. He may give up and resort to his previous eating habits. If he continues his old habits, major problems will occur.

Diabetic menus, exchange lists and food values are not as difficult to understand as some would have you believe. It has been said, attitude is a wonderful thing, if it is the "right attitude." Successful diabetics have proved the truth of this statement, relative to their approach to diabetic control.

Many scientists, doctors and dieticians have worked for many years, independently and together, searching out the most easily understood diabetic diet, and the best way to apply it.

Each diet is designed to be very palatable and varied, and for this, every diabetic should be thankful.

The first lesson to learn about the diet, is to keep it simple. It is much easier to calculate and measure the uncomplicated foods.

It is natural to see how many eye-pleasing and palate-pleasing dishes can be created, and still stay within the limits of the diet.

Too often, the diabetic discovers that the involved preparation becomes a burden, and because he is not familiar with food values, he begins to feel like an octopus, tangled in his own tentacles. This should never happen.

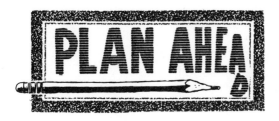

It is wise to plan meals one day in advance, for then you will be sure that all food and ingredients are available. Don't say to yourself, "I think there is asparagus in the freezer," and a few minutes before mealtime, discover there is none. It may happen at the same time, that you are out of other vegetables, as well. Insulin won't wait for you to "run to the store."

Try to avoid the pressure of last minute preparation. All cooks know how LITTLE complications can slip in at the last moment. The diabetic cook has difficulty resolving a crowded situation, and must avoid panic, at all cost.

One reason that diabetics experience difficulty just before a meal, is that often the blood sugar has dropped just enough to cause nervousness and jitteriness, not otherwise noted. Planning ahead, keeping calm and eating food as promptly as possible, combine to form the antidote.

If you are employed, be sure to get up in the morning in ample time to eat a complete breakfast. If you carry a lunch, allow adequate time to prepare it. Never leave the house without having eaten a complete breakfast, and carry with you, a complete lunch.

It is best not to rely on indefinite plans, such as, "I'll drop into Joe's place and pick up something." You may get there too late and also, he may not have what you require at the time you need it.

It is well to remember that diabetics cannot skip or delay a meal. An unscheduled snack may throw the control off completely. This is not good diabetic planning.

Foods are calculated, either by measurement or weight. Freedom from the scale has come to many diabetics within the last few years. However, many of the severe diabetics must continue with the gram scale program. The mild diabetic, as a rule, can measure his food, and experience adequate control.

When the "amount" of food is limited, the "choice" of food becomes extremely important. By varying the food, the body has the opportunity to absorb the many body building ingredients it needs.

Volume of food is not the answer to satisfying the appetite. A balanced diet is. If you continue to be hungry, you may not be adhering to the diet as prescribed by the doctor.

Often, we hear patients in the hospital, say something like this, "I've lost 8 pounds this week, and wasn't a bit hungry." There are thousands of instances like this, which prove what a BALANCED diet can do!

When the diabetic controls his appetite and stays with the prescribed diet, his sense of well-being increases. Also, when his weight is excessive, he must reduce it, and living within the limit of the diet, will help him to accomplish this. Doctors tell us that normal weight brings improved health and decreases the severity of diabetes. Avoid obesity! *(More on this later.)*

A neighbor once said, "My husband is a diabetic, and we can never keep baked goods, or anything like it, in our house. My husband eats it before we do!" Of course, this is a selfish, and childish attitude of an uncontrolled diabetic. Let ALL diabetics stay away from this kind of frustrated living.

On the other hand, the wife of another diabetic, said, "Ever since my husband became diabetic, my daughter and I are eating the same diet as my husband. We both feel so much better!" She continued, "And look," as she turned around proudly, "I'm now my correct weight. Isn't it wonderful?" Everyone admired her for this, especially as they recalled her unsuccessful attempts at reducing.

This type of adjustment in living is perfect, and every diabetic household would do well to follow her example.

Again, select and measure (or weigh) your food, put everything else out of sight and mind. ENJOY WHAT YOU HAVE, AND FORGET WHAT YOU CANNOT HAVE.

Many diabetics who have difficulty in achieving control, have discovered that saving the fruit from breakfast, and eating it two or three hours later, helps them to reduce the sugar level at breakfast time. Also, it carries them over a period during the morning, which may be one of being too sugar free.

The same may be done with the evening meal. The fruit could serve as a snack before retiring. Half of the milk allowed at the evening meal, could also be saved and enjoyed with the fruit.

This relieves the strain of digestion at mealtime and helps to cover a drop in the blood sugar, during the night.

BE SURE TO CHECK BOTH OF THESE IDEAS WITH YOUR DOCTOR. If the doctor approves such a program, special care must be taken to eat this food at the scheduled hour. Otherwise, the omitted carbohydrate, essential in balancing the insulin taken earlier, may precipitate an insulin reaction. This, the diabetic does not want.

It has been suggested that milk and butter may be measured for the day, in advance. One meal may call for more of each than another. When the "measured-out" amount is gone, you know "that's it for that day."

If you still have dinner to prepare, you may be in difficulty. As soon as the diabetic understands this, he will save adequate milk and fat ingredients for cooking.

Too much fat in the diet, hastens undesired complications. Those in research tell us that the polyunsaturated fats such as margarines, low calorie cooking oils, et cetera, are permissible and sometimes preferable for the diabetic's use. Be sure to check this point with your doctor also, as every diabetic has individual needs.

The artificial sweeteners on the market are abundant. These products are not harmful to health. How thankful all diabetics should be for this!

There are now literally hundreds of foods available, prepared with the sugarless sweeteners. This has opened a great variety of foods for the diabetic to enjoy. These many varieties of food are available in most stores, and may be found in a special section designated for them.

As a rule, the food values are printed on the package. Be sure to read them carefully.

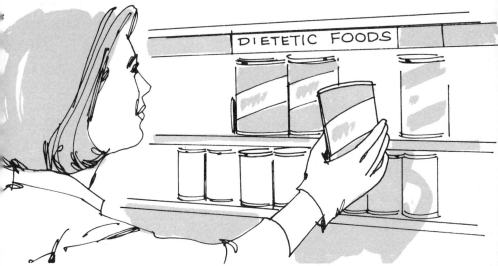

Also, be SURE you understand the food value of a product BEFORE using it. Don't be satisfied with the advice of someone else. Also, take note of the number of calories it contains. The product may look harmless, and the advertising may sound very inviting, but the diabetic cannot take chances.

Sometime ago, Jolene saw a product that read "No sugar or salt added." It looked so inviting, that without reading further, she took some home, and that evening, included two of the small harmless looking biscuits in her diet. They were delicious!

So she included two at lunch, also. After a few days, the scale "lifted its brow" when she stepped on it, for she had gained four pounds.

Reviewing her food intake again, the four little biscuits were suspected. By reading the fine print on the package, it was revealed that each little biscuit contained 95 calories! The food she had substituted them for contained only 60 calories. So each day, she was adding 320 calories.

While the sugarless foods on the market are a great asset, do make sure to read the calorie contents before using them.

When control was placed in the hands of the diabetic, he had to accept the responsibility for learning food values, the weighing of food by grams, and learning the art of making substitutions in the diet, while still retaining the proper amounts of carbohydrates, proteins, fats and calories.

Today, this task is greatly simplified, through the use of classified charts.

An excellent chart, making easy the method of breaking down the caloric intake, and foods to correct measurement, has been produced by The Upjohn Company of Kalamazoo, Michigan. The chart is entitled "Calorie Control For You," and was developed from "Meal Planning With Exchange Lists" by committees from The American Diabetes Association and The American Dietetic Association.

This chart has been produced in several languages by The Upjohn Company, and if you wish to obtain one of them, it is suggested you consult your doctor and he will secure it for you, or he may suggest that you write the company direct.

Your doctor will circle the correct caloric level for you. The diabetic simply follows the number of servings from each list, designated to meet the caloric intake. The exchange lists are included on the chart.

As a rule, we seldom think of water as a food, but in reality it is a very important one. Diabetics are constantly reminded to drink an adequate amount of water. Because the original uncontrollable thirst disappears when control with insulin is obtained, drinking water, is often overlooked and even forgotten.

The kidneys love to work, and for the diabetic, the elimination of waste through the kidneys is extremely important, and water does perform this function.

PLEASE NOTE

When purchasing dry cereals, be sure to eliminate the sugar coated varieties.

Fresh, frozen, canned or cooked fruits and vegetables may be used. However, if any of these are processed with sugar, choose another brand.

Canned fruit juice, without sugar added, has the same food value as the fresh. The concentrated fruit juice, processed without sugar, has the same food value as the fresh, AFTER WATER HAS BEEN ADDED according to directions on the can.

Plain gelatin and sugar-free gelatin desserts, have no food value and may be used as desired.

SOME SWEETS TO THE SWEET

One of the misconceptions prevalent today, is that diabetics cannot eat sugar. It must be remembered that no matter what kind or form of carbohydrates we eat, ALL carbohydrates turn to sugar, when they are digested.

The diabetic needs carbohydrates to balance the insulin with proteins and fats. Fruits, vegetables, breads and cereals are excellent sources of carbohydrates, and work well to bring about this balance.

The diabetic's diet is based on his age, height, weight, occupation, exercise, sex and the severity of his condition.

When the doctor works out this diet, he keeps all of these considerations in mind, and each diabetic is wise to follow the doctor's prescriptions.

Every diabetic should memorize his list of foods, so that the selection of food is easier. Also, when visiting away from home, or traveling, he will be able to substitute foods without difficulty. He will find, that his close association with foods, will help him to build his knowledge and the use of foods.

Usually, it is best for the diabetic to eat at home. He knows what he needs, and what is available! At home, he has the best control of the timing and amount of food involved. Diabetics have learned that it pays to eat at home, and attend social functions later in the evening.

A fellow diabetic said to Jolene, "How is your appetite?" She replied, "Oh, fine. I just keep whittling away at it." He smiled with understanding. All diabetics realize there is quite a difference between hunger and appetite.

Appetite makes all food desirous, hunger makes us satisfied with what we get. Your appetite may always be good, but a diabetic is seldom very hungry. Let us today, be grateful for the food we are privileged to enjoy, because of insulin control and the use of oral compounds.

It is a good idea to do your food shopping as soon AFTER a meal as possible. You won't be as tempted to buy something you know, should be left in the store.

Oh, yes, diabetics should eat slowly. Doctors tell us there is a definite advantage, as the food is assimilated much better.

NO SHARING OF FOOD

A diabetic should never give his food away, no matter what the circumstances may be. He can't afford to short-change himself.

Jolene Jordan had an experience of this kind not long ago. She had taken her lunch to the office, which covered only her own needs. A former employee dropped in with her baby girl for a visit. When the little girl saw Jolene's banana, her eyes were big. Jolene tried not to notice it, as she knew she would be in trouble if she omitted this food.

Another employee spoke up and said, "Jolene, I think some-one wants your banana." Jolene cut off a small piece of it and gave it to the little girl. This did not suffice, and her longing eyes almost broke Jolene's heart.

Jolene had no choice, and amidst the disapproving eyes of co-workers and the disappointed eyes of a little child, she had to eat the banana. To this day, Jolene thinks of this, every time she eats a banana.

Another experience came one day when Jolene forgot to take her lunch along. Remembering it in mid-morning, she left the office to go home to get it. Just then another girl said, "Oh, don't do that, Jolene, I have an extra sandwhich with me today, and will be happy to give it to you."

Because she insisted, Jolene accepted and was grateful. But the following day, Jolene again took her regular lunch, which again only covered her own need, and the friend from the day before, said immediately, "I forgot my lunch today, could you help me out?"

Jolene was caught again unexpectedly, but it taught her to stay away from food obligations, and this, she has managed to do.

It is imperative that the diabetic assume all responsibility concerning the management of his diabetes at home. This includes selection, measuring (or weighing) food, timing, et cetera. Rely only on yourself for these controls.

Never feel your "guesstimate" is as good as measuring or weighing. It's strange, how quickly the amount YOU take, can increase. If someone ELSE is giving it to you, he is apt to decrease the amount. Neither is good.

In conclusion, diabetics are truly grateful to doctors and dieticians for their conscientious work in establishing proper food control. They also appreciate their dedication to the art of teaching this very important subject of food, to them.

FOR WEIGHTS, MEASURES, CALORIES AND SUCH,
WE THANK YOU ALL, SO VERY MUCH!

* * * * * * * *

Elsewhere in this book, you will find the suggestion to subscribe to the bimonthly magazine, ADA FORECAST, published by the American Diabetes Association.

If you are not a subscriber now, become one, for this magazine will become your "cup of tea."

It is helpful to the diabetic in the area of understanding and the preparation of a diabetic menu.

In 1959 the American Diabetes Association published the *Cookbook for Diabetics* which was a collection of SISTER MAUDE's recipes and directions written through the years. It is an outstanding work of its kind and has achieved a distribution of over 425,000 copies. It is a very significant contribution to the education of diabetics which sprung from the pen, the mind and the heart of SISTER MAUDE.

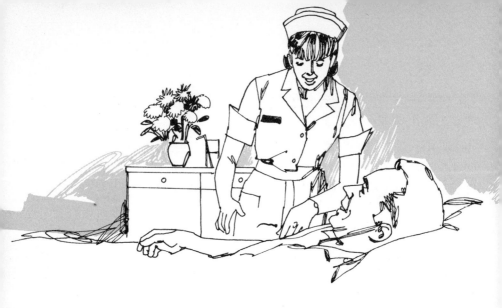

THE DIABETIC'S HOSPITAL

When the hospital admits a diabetic, the staff realizes that here is a patient with special and exacting needs.

No matter what illness may bring the diabetic to the hospital, he always brings with him, his diabetes.

There may be no other illness where the patient needs to be informed of his treatment as much as does the diabetic. Doctors, nurses, in fact, all hospital staff members, are aware of this.

The patient is informed of his food intake, timing, insulin needs and general information about his control. His history "at home" also becomes an important factor in the treatment at the hospital.

Here then, is still another good reason for the diabetic to maintain daily, yes—hourly, control at home, for it is only then that he has the ability to provide helpful information to the hospital staff.

Hospital personnel find it works well, to begin treatment where the patient left off, and keep the routine as near to the patient's "at home" procedure as possible. They know any drastic departure from the diabetic's schedule could upset him to the point of uncontrollability, and complicate the ailment for which he was hospitalized.

Of course, the diabetic must again assume the control at the end of his hospital stay, therefore, he must be informed of all results, such as the urine tests, the amount and kind of insulin used.

He must fully understand about the food intake as prescribed by the doctor, analyzed and produced by the dietician, as well as the results of other tests like blood sugar, blood pressure, blood count, et cetera.

Because he has this information, he feels more confident when he assumes control at home, because of the intelligent and educational reporting by, and discussions with, professional personnel.

For this reason, all hospital personnel seek to work with the patient's "at home" experience, in order to help him be better fortified when he returns home.

A diabetic woman once said, "Everytime a hospital-nurse gives me insulin she checks my name, the doctor's name, and tells me the amount and kind of insulin she is about to give me. Is all that necessary?"

Yes, every nurse is trained to do this and wisely secures this confirmation from the patient BEFORE giving the insulin. This method prevents mistakes. Insulin is serious business. It is not a sedative.

Be grateful for a cautious nurse. She has the role of being teacher and counsellor, to help you with the "exacting" care you must always take with insulin injections.

This education in the hospital is important and every question you ask and every answer you receive, will help to insure better control, when you arrive at home.

If the patient is a new diabetic, the hospital is one of the best places to learn how to make tests, to understand about the kind of insulin prescribed, the syringe and how to read it, how to draw out the insulin and prevent bubbles from appearing in the syringe, how to combine insulins in the same dosage, if more than one kind is taken, and how to keep a daily record sheet. This education of the diabetic may necessitate a longer stay in the hospital than would otherwise be called for.

Hospital care can be a haven for the diabetic. As a rule, diabetics need extra rest, and their stay in the hospital should cause them to feel relaxed, as it is perhaps the only opportunity they have to lie down, and feel life will continue. All patients are given the opportunity to rest and recover.

The patient must always cooperate completely with the hospital personnel. A diabetic woman, in the hospital, was observed to be running high sugar, over which her doctor was puzzled and was trying to find the explanation. Her roommate noted that each evening her daughter brought a pint of ice cream and two bottles of soda pop, which they enjoyed "party-style." Need more be said?

HELPS IN HOSPITAL LIVING

While in the hospital, telephone calls should be kept at a minimum. Some patients have been known to discuss their illness, the doctor's latest remarks, each test in detail, as well as their life's problems, past, present and possible future solutions. This can become very annoying and upsetting to the roommate, as well as to busy nurses.

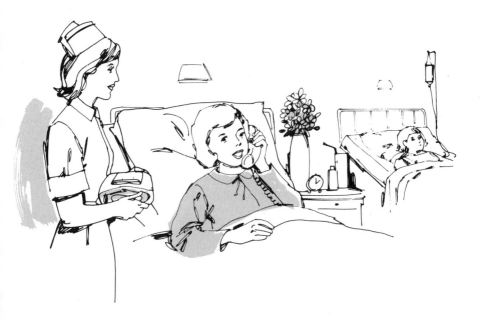

Can you imagine having the nurse wait to give a bath and change the linens, while the patient tells Aunt Betty all the things her husband failed to get done the day before? This is very inconsiderate, and should never be allowed to happen. Calls should be kept to a minimum. Cooperation is essential.

Keep visitors to a minimum. Visitors to a diabetic, are not able to know or choose the best time for calling. The diabetic's time is quite consumed with tests, injections, food, and both the personnel and the patient agree that too much company interferes.

A bright "card" with a friendly note, does more for the diabetic, than phone calls and visitors. Jolene remembers with a warm heart, a Valentine's Day she spent in the hospital when a card shower was sent by fellow workers from her office.

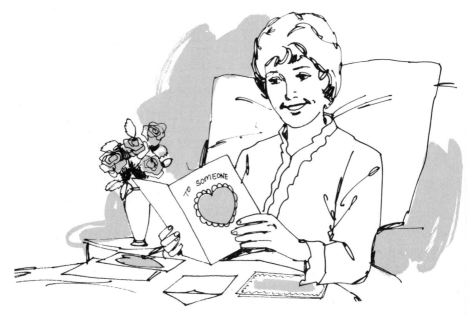

Some were humorous which raised her spirits, others were warm and sincere which made her very happy. Each one had a personal note which meant much more to her than if the friends had telephoned or come in person. Each additional time she read them, was like another visit.

Here are a couple of helpful "don'ts."

Don't talk about your illness all the time.
Don't encourage your roommate to talk about his/her ill-
ness either.

This does neither one any good, and some may find it emotionally difficult to listen to a constant stream of detailed accounts of illnesses, usually coupled with complaints.

The importance of a diabetic getting adequate sleep and rest, while in the hospital, cannot be over emphasized. He may survive one or even two nights of interrupted rest, but by the third night it takes its toll and begins to reflect itself in his control.

The more calm a diabetic can remain while in the hospital, the speedier his recovery.

When a diabetic becomes ill, there is no better place for him to be, than in the hospital. Every patient is grateful for the watchful care, the teaching and counselling, he receives.

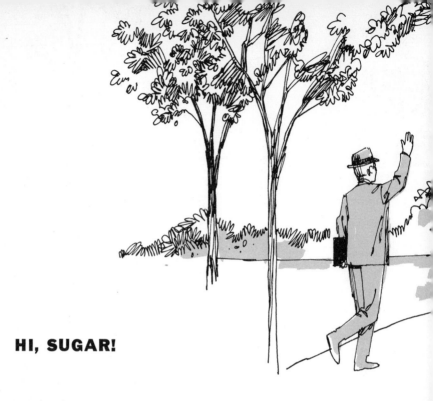

HI, SUGAR!

My husband calls me pet names.
And I love them, every one.
But here's the one, I like the best.
For with it, we have fun—
    "HI, SUGAR!"

He knows his diabetes,
(Though he's never studied medics,)
He joins me now in greeting YOU
And ALL the diabetics—
    "HI, SUGAR!"

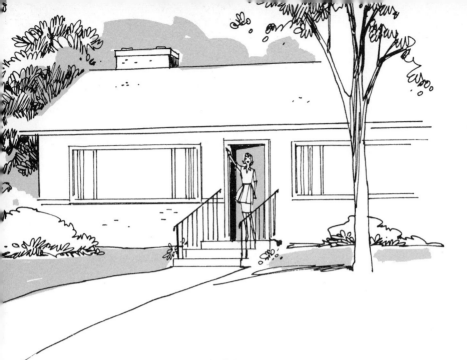

THE ART OF LIVING

It has been pointed out that the first responsibility of successful diabetic living, belongs to the patient.

Now, let's consider the responsibilities of his family, his friends, employer and co-workers. Their attitude can make or break the diabetic.

Since these folk are very important to every diabetic, each member of this group needs to understand how he can contribute to make life normal and enjoyable' for the diabetic.

While this total social circle has many "common" approaches, each group has specific considerations which are peculiar to its own group. Let's see how this works out.

THE FAMILY

Living with diabetes within the family is not always easy, because it must be remembered that each member of the family has his own interests.

However, consideration FOR the diabetic and HIS problems should come first, and at the same time, the demanding and important requirements of ALL members of the family should not be overlooked.

Adjustments need to be made to incorporate all phases of family living. If each member is willing to swing as far as he can, to meet the needs of the other, then it is possible to solve all family problems. This leads to successful diabetic family living.

Perhaps the first step towards this congenial family living is the omission of frequent discussions on diabetes. A general interest in the diabetic and his control is vital, especially by the husband or wife. If the diabetic is a child, then both parents should carry this responsibility and this interest.

It would appear, however, that the only necessary discussion in the home on diabetes, is the training involved, the interest in test results, the amount of insulin taken and the questions which may arise about food intake.

These expressions of interest are necessary, but long and labored discussions are not. This approach will leave plenty of time for other interests and activities.

Some folk take on the role of judge and jury and make the diabetic's life more difficult. If he is guilty of eating food that is not in his diet, he will realize it, on his own.

"Nagging" only increases his frustration and may start an emotional ball of resentment rolling, which the diabetic and the family may find difficult to control.

A trusted diabetic is a happy diabetic. He may have good reasons for eating extra food, and having to prove his need for it, only adds to his problem.

Yes, he knows the score better than anyone else, and interference does not help, it only hinders.

As a family member, remember this, the diabetic is growing daily in his approach to adequate control and you must grow with him. Your silence may be much more effective than your word of caution, and your smile more effective than your reprimand.

There is the story about the diabetic husband who was nagged by his wife about food, insulin and testing, so—he dipped the Tes-Tape in pure water and displayed a "sugar-free" test—to still her tongue. What a price he paid for peace! Before long, HIS tongue was stilled forever.

If the diabetic does break his diet either through ignorance or carelessness, there is no one more sorry for having broken faith with you, with himself and his doctor, than the diabetic himself.

He suffers conscience pangs which you will never know. A diabetic is a human being. He is not a robot, nor a "pin cushion" that has no feelings. He is a person with courage and a conscience, treat him with kindness and understanding.

It seems every family has at least one "medical advisor." This can be trying, even fatal. The judgment of the advisor is based on what he "heard" or "read" or "thought he saw." He may say, with horror in his eyes, "You're eating an orange! Don't you know oranges have sugar in them?" Little does he realize that oranges are the life-line food for the diabetic, taking insulin.

The diet of a diabetic is not too different from a normal diet, and everyone should be educated to this fact. We have often heard, a little knowledge is dangerous, and this is also true in the case of the family medical advisor. Do be careful!

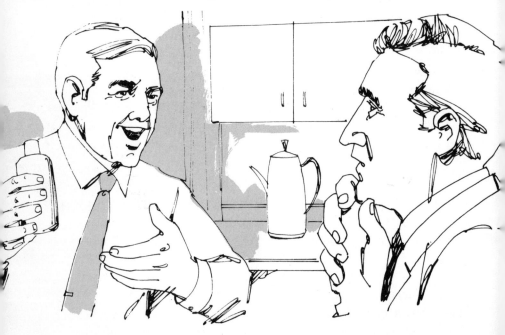

Then, there is the family "pill-pusher." Articles are read by family members on the value of certain medications for the diabetic, and immediately a crusade is begun to start the diabetic on these drugs.

Here is a very important fact to remember, and should be written deep in the mind and heart of every diabetic, with capital letters:

▶ A DIABETIC SHOULD NEVER TAKE ANY MEDICA-TION, UNLESS IT IS PRESCRIBED BY HIS DOCTOR!

Ask your doctor for his opinion on ANY medication, for this is the ONLY way he can carry the responsibility for your care. Remember, the well-intentioned family pill-pusher and family advisor can NEVER be permitted to replace the doctor.

The diabetic must maintain his independence concerning his care at home. Don't permit a family member to get the education about your illness and expect him to carry the responsibility for your care. Remember YOU are the one who will need that knowledge and experience as long as YOU live.

It is impossible for a lazy diabetic to be a successful diabetic. If you have a tendency toward letting someone else carry the responsibility for your control, then get busy and change that attitude right away. You will find more happiness and self-satisfaction than you ever dreamed possible.

Thank you, Dr. Joslin, for your manual on diabetes, and for these words which have been repeated many times silently within Jolene's diabetic heart:

"He who learns and learns,
Yet does not what he knows,
Is one who plows and plows
Yet, never sows."

*(Translated from the Persian by
James Phinney Baster)*

The diabetic must learn all he can about diabetes, and USE this knowledge to improve his control and general well-being.

The diabetic is wise to schedule medical appointments, shopping tours, social visits, et cetera, so they do not interfere with his diabetic schedule.

He should return home in ample time to prepare a meal and eat. Always consider that a shopping trip, plus carrying packages, involves extra exercise. and may present the need for an earlier meal.

With early detection and adequate control, family living with diabetes is normal. Again, play it cool, avoid tenseness, and remember, cheerfulness is the best antidote for family complications.

THE FRIENDS

There is a general opinion, that diabetics seek seclusion and have introversial tendencies. This is not so. Diabetics, as a rule, are extroversial, outgoing, friendly people. They do have restrictions on food and time of course, which must get priority at all times. This fact is not always understood.

When friends or relatives call a diabetic on the phone, their first question should be, "Do you have time to talk now, or should I call later?"

If the diabetic has just taken insulin, or the insulin taken several hours earlier, is beginning to climax, and he is preparing to eat, it is unwise to take the time for a lengthy telephone conversation.

The diabetic should offer to call back or specify the time for the friend to call. Insulin does not wait, but most phone conversations can. If the message is urgent, then give it as quickly as possible and hang up, without delay.

This same thoughtfulness should exist when making social calls. The habit of "dropping in" on a diabetic should be eliminated. Diabetics are delighted with family and friends, but phone calls and visits must be planned.

Jolene Jordan can well recall the evening she took regular insulin and five minutes later, guests dropped in for a visit. Of course, regular insulin calls for food within 15 to 30 minutes.

There was not enough time to prepare for guests, and there was nothing else to do, but to tell her friends the situation and ask them to return at some other time. Their next visit was well planned.

One of the first lessons for friends and relatives to learn, is that a diabetic must keep a close schedule. If you are invited by a diabetic host or hostess, be sure to arrive at the appointed hour.

If your diabetic hostess calmly serves you and then sits down unflustered to eat, respect her. She has planned ahead to accomplish this. It didn't just happen that way!

Very often, friends expect too much from the diabetic. He may look well, but he may have a feeling of inner weakness. He does not want to admit this to himself, much less, to others.

After a good day's work, a diabetic must have a good night's sleep. It would be wonderful, if friends could understand why the diabetic does not always do things they expect. Understanding friends can do much for the diabetic's inward tranquility.

If the diabetic is disturbed by someone, and the situation cannot be straightened out, then he should not hesitate to put a great distance between himself and the offender. He cannot afford to indulge in irregular or strenuous living.

A new diabetic tries hard to incorporate all of the old activities, but soon finds he has to make a choice in favor of healthful living.

Friends are fun and diabetics need and enjoy them all. The greatest gift a friend can give the diabetic is this understanding. Constantly discussing the diabetes is NO help.

Permitting the diabetic to decide what he can and cannot do, without having to prove his point, is a tremendous help.

BUILD ON THE OLD FRIENDSHIP, BY ADDING NEW UNDERSTANDING, THEREBY DEVELOPING A GREATER HELPFULNESS TO THE DIABETIC!

EMPLOYERS AND CO-WORKERS

While at work, the diabetic carries full responsibility for his control. He must, therefore, know his condition at all times.

If he is driving a car, he must make sure that his control is adequate for each trip. He should always start in plenty of time, anticipating problems of delay.

Also, while at work, he should drink plenty of water. This important requirement of diabetic living is often overlooked or forgotten while at work. The cold fountains and interest in his work combine to cause the omission of this detail.

Research has turned up a few observations that will be an encouragement to both, the worker and the employer.

The health of a diabetic is not in jeopardy when employed. In fact, it is a great help to him.

The diabetic is an excellent employee. We are told most diabetics are in the higher mental calibre range and are efficient workers.

The diabetic is faithful and conscientious. The self-discipline of his control, pays off in many ways.

His attendance is regular.
His disposition is cheerful and cooperative.
His loyalty to the company is strong.
He loves to work.

Now, on the other hand, his health will become affected, when the atmosphere at work is unhappy, or unpleasantness occurs within the company. This is one reason, each diabetic strives hard to keep the day pleasant. Congeniality and harmony spell success for the working diabetic.

The emotional structure of a diabetic is such that he cannot tolerate anything but tranquil surroundings. When arguments, unkind remarks and attitudes develop, even though the diabetic is not personally involved, he may as well pack his pencils and seek more peaceful surroundings.

It is a known fact, that many fine employees have been lost to companies, because the employer and co-workers did not understand this very vivid problem of the diabetic.

It is unfortunate, when co-workers seek out the subject of diabetes at coffee breaks, lunches, social gatherings or private conversations, when they know there is a diabetic present.

Often they ask many questions and then discount the answers. There is at least one person who likes to relate over and over some unpleasant story which has been brought down through the family, from the dark days before insulin.

Also, the diabetic often cannot enjoy his food, without someone saying, "Can YOU have THAT?"

Frequently, there are unkind people who use diabetes as a wedge to try and influence the thinking of the powers that be, to turn a decision against the diabetic, because of his illness.

The enlarged thinking about diabetes and the knowledge concerning the improved living conditions and life expectancy, have not become as well known as they might. The diabetic is often dealt with, unfairly and the truth is not known. Many diabetics today are suffering from such situations, and this is sad.

When diabetics seek employment, they do tell the Personnel Director and their immediate superior of their condition. Beyond this, they usually do not wish to discuss their problems.

Not because they are trying to hide it, and there certainly is no stigma attached, but they have discovered that others can't seem to drop the subject.

Diabetics are, as a rule, active people, who enjoy conversations on interesting topics. Co-workers could help greatly by omitting the undesirable discussion on diabetes, and thereby create a much happier spirit for effective and cooperative business relations.

When these important phases of diabetic living are considered, he is better able to live with his restrictions and enjoy his life, his work, and the people around him.

It is well for everyone to remember, diabetics inherited the illness, through no fault of their own. Respect them, when they try to control it.

The diabetic's health, and eventually his life, are at stake. Can there be a better reason to help him?

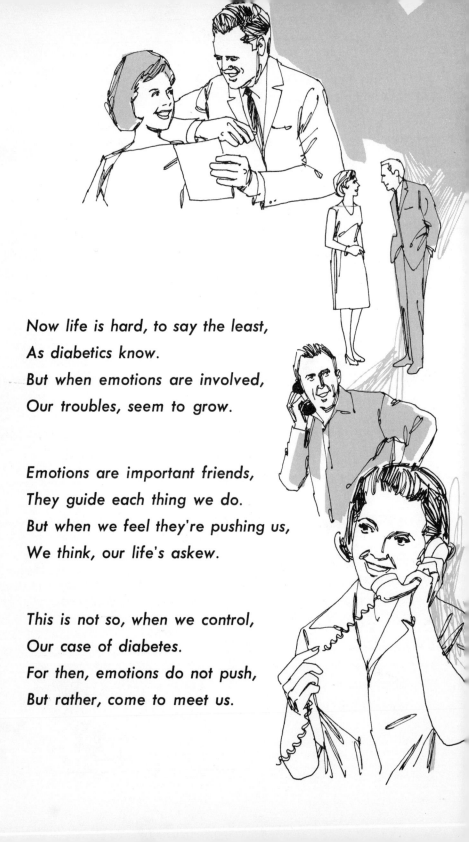

Now life is hard, to say the least,
As diabetics know.
But when emotions are involved,
Our troubles, seem to grow.

Emotions are important friends,
They guide each thing we do.
But when we feel they're pushing us,
We think, our life's askew.

This is not so, when we control,
Our case of diabetes.
For then, emotions do not push,
But rather, come to meet us.

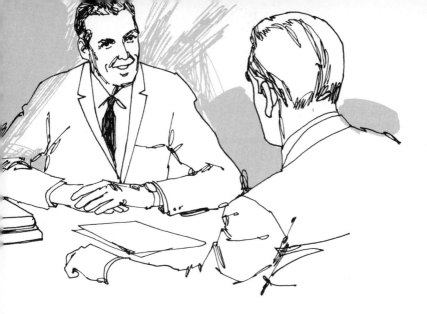

SWEET EMOTIONS

Everyone is born with emotions, and they are a part of our personalities and environment.

Controlled emotions is something of which we may be proud. It is strange, however, the stigma that is so often attached to the word "emotions."

It is true, there are good emotions and some not so good, but all of them need to be controlled, to produce what we call a "stable" man or a "stable" woman.

When emotions, controlled or uncontrolled, are combined with diabetes, something happens to the inner framework of the diabetic.

We are told, diabetes affects the nervous system, and it is believed this is the reason the emotions are so deeply involved. The more complicated the case of diabetes, the more complicated the emotions.

As control of the diabetes increases, the emotions level off, and the diabetic discovers a new inner strength. This control, as always, is the result of combining insulin, food, testing and exercise. This then, is the balanced living, all diabetics aspire to, and must achieve.

The diabetic must also have a doctor who understands the problem, one who has much experience, maturity and a personality that creates confidence within the diabetic.

The diabetic's understanding of his own condition, the confidence in his control, instilled by the doctor, and the encouragement and cooperation of his family and friends, are the greatest stabilizers of emotions, known to the diabetic.

It is a known fact that "depression" is one emotion that arrives at the same time as diabetes, but this too, vanishes, when control is adequate. These fragile emotions, which play such an important role in the diabetic's daily living, must be recognized and overcome.

Very often a diabetic will accept blame before he will permit himself to become involved in an emotional problem.

Jolene can well recall several instances in her experience, when she was accused of something that was untrue, but took the blame without answering, because she knew her emotions would fail her, if she tried to defend herself.

This creates unfair treatment and the integrity of the diabetic is often in question, because he doesn't dare indulge in argument, discussion or nervous strain of any kind.

Remember this:

IN AN EMOTIONAL UPSET, ALL INSULIN
ACTION IN THE BODY—CEASES!

This is something to think about. An emotional upset does not necessarily mean it must be major, before it affects the insulin action. Some minor irritation throughout the day, or worry, can cause the same difficulty in control.

The diabetic cannot do anything about the onset of these side effects, but there are many very important ways the diabetic can intercept their progress, and keep the destruction to a minimum. The most important way is to keep the diabetes under as perfect a control as possible. CONTROL IS YOUR GREATEST SOLUTION!

If the diabetic finds himself in an unbearable situation, it behooves him either to resolve the problem, assume another attitude, or change the situation to one of compatibility. These are hard, cold facts to face, but harder yet to accept and live with, daily.

Jolene says, "Every successful diabetic I have known, seems to be adjusted and equal to the task of every-day-diabetic-living, and is cheerful, despite the fact that he lives under certain rules and restrictions." It is precisely this attitude, which is responsible for his success.

One woman commented and also asked, "My husband is a diabetic and he is always irritable. Are all diabetics irritable?" The answer was, "No, certainly not."

If a diabetic is "well controlled," there is no reason for a continuous irritability.

Often, an inner weakness, which diabetics sometimes feel, but do not mention, or a brief time of being too sugar-free, may cause a temporary irritable reaction. These conditions are never sustained.

There are many strange and erroneous beliefs which cause people to harrass the diabetic today. These opinions come from the old days prior to insulin, and against which he must constantly battle. Here are some of them.

YOU GET DIABETES FROM OVEREATING SWEETS

This is not true. Food plays no part in "acquiring" the condition, but plays a major role in controlling it. Jolene Jordan knows, that if the former were true, she would not have diabetes. She was too "figure conscious" at the age, she became diabetic. Diabetes is hereditary.

ONCE YOU GET DIABETES, IT IS ALWAYS SEVERE

This also is not true. Many people have shown sugar in the urine at the time of some special stress, may at that time be diagnosed as diabetic, but when the problems subsided, the sugar disappeared. Some diagnosed diabetics have been known to recover completely, but this is rare.

When severe diabetes is controlled with insulin and diet, the case may become mild, and mild cases with treatment, can sometimes be controlled with an oral compound or diet alone.

WHEN YOU BECOME DIABETIC, LIFE IS OVER

This is completely untrue, and it hurts to write such a heading. Before insulin, figuratively speaking, the black crepe was hung on the door at the time of diagnosis. But now, with the use of insulin, *and let's say it again, a diabetic can look forward to a full and normal span of life.*

Doctors report that diabetics, as a rule, have an unusually high IQ. They are conscientious workers, are happy individuals and they are sympathetic with others, who have the same or other illnesses.

And life is not over for the diabetic child either. Thousands of them have grown into well adjusted adults, achieved success in their chosen fields and become a source of pride to their families and the medical profession.

DIABETES CAUSES OTHER ILLNESSES

Again, this is not true. A diabetic is like other people. He is susceptible to other illnesses, but because he has diabetes, does not necessarily mean he is more vulnerable to other illnesses. Of course, this applies to the "controlled" diabetic. What a great responsibility each diabetic carries!

DIABETICS GO BLIND, LOSE FOOT OR LEG

This is absolutely not true. Recently, Jolene overheard a woman say, "We stopped to visit Alice yesterday. She is diabetic, and of course almost blind."

This statement cut through Jolene's heart, for once again the feeling was expressed that if you are diabetic, you are going blind. Not so!

It is true that diabetes, over a period of years, affects the arteries throughout the body, including the eyes and extremities. If the diabetic maintains good control every day, his chances of developing these complications are minimized. The well controlled diabetic, after many years, sometimes develops these problems. Knowing this fact, should help all diabetics to see to it that his daily control is complete.

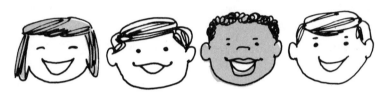

THE BRIGHT SIDE OF EMOTIONS

Again, cheerfulness in the well adjusted diabetic, will help him and his family to live in harmony. The experience of most diabetics is that the family is willing to meet them, more than halfway.

After a diabetic has mastered the various steps of his daily routine, he must shake "from himself," all thought "of himself." He should direct his efforts to interest in others, and into a full and rewarding life for himself.

He will then become confident that his knowledge and the rigid application of it, will ease the emotional tension for himself and his family, and through this approach, prolong his life.

He will know in his heart, that he is doing his best, and if, in later years some misfortune should befall him, he can always feel, it was not the result of neglect.

What a comfort this one thought alone should be to the diabetic and his loved ones!

Diabetics should ALWAYS remember the bright side of their condition. Here are some shining examples:

Diabetes is controllable.
Diabetes is not painful.
Diabetes does not deform.
Diabetes is not contagious.
Diabetic diets are full and complete, and very palatable.
Diabetic diets build up resistance and prevent other illnesses.
Diabetics are not bedridden.
Diabetics are mentally alert.
Diabetics are active, working people.

When one stops to consider the many benefits "controlled" diabetics enjoy today, the few limitations and "musts" fade into the background.

APPRECIATE EVERY "PLUS" YOUR DIABETIC CONDITION HAS BROUGHT YOU, AND THINK OF EVERY "MINUS" AS SOMETHING TO FORGET!

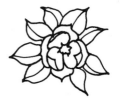

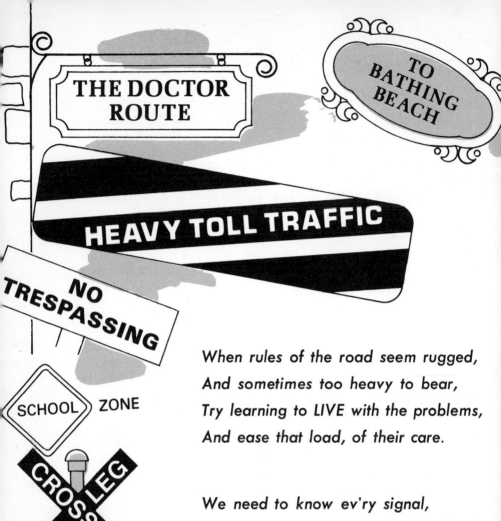

THE DOCTOR ROUTE

TO BATHING BEACH

HEAVY TOLL TRAFFIC

NO TRESPASSING

SCHOOL ZONE

NO LEG CROSSING

When rules of the road seem rugged,
And sometimes too heavy to bear,
Try learning to LIVE with the problems,
And ease that load, of their care.

We need to know ev'ry signal,
We need to know ev'ry chart,
And if we OBEY each warning,
New strength, flows into our heart.

If we learn these rules, that will help us,
Live by them, every day.
We find that we walk much better,
Through life's diabetic way.

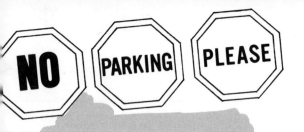

SIGNPOSTS on the DIABETIC ROAD

We have been warned many times, when driving the family car over the country's highways, to "Drive as if our lives depended upon it."

When traveling on the diabetic road, we can do no less. Whether we are a new or an experienced traveler, we need to know the rules of the road. Yes, our continued activities, even our very lives, depend upon reading and heeding the signposts along the way.

If each diabetic could look ahead 20, 40 or 60 years, and see the havoc "uncontrolled" diabetes can cause, he would then carefully check the signposts, absorb the rules and heed them.

He must always remember, as he travels the diabetic road each day, that he owes his very best living to his family, doctor, employer, friends, insurance company, and the public in general. Last, but far from least, he owes it to himself.

Here are a few of the signposts put up to guide the diabetic and those around him, to DECREASE the diabetic problems, and INCREASE the happiness he and others will experience through controlled living, while traveling that diabetic road.

THE DOCTOR ROUTE

Secure a good doctor, one with whom you feel compatible, and cooperate with him. Keep your visits to his office on a regular and punctual basis.

Upon each visit, take with you a complete record of your test results, amount of insulin taken, and your diet, covering the time since you last saw him.

It is a "must" that the doctor know exactly what you are doing to achieve control, whether you are adequately successful, or, if changes are necessary.

Here are a few of the records, your doctor will appreciate:

Keeping alert to the over-all condition.
Recording all additional medication.
Noting time of reactions, and antidote used.
Observing acetone occurrences.
Recording all of the food intake, and adjustments.

These records will help as a reference for the future. A solution to the present problem, may be found in the record of the past.

The busy doctor will appreciate this complete report, and at a glance will recognize the problems and successes. It will eliminate the extra time required for verbal reporting.

ROUTE ALL YOUR PROBLEMS THROUGH
THE DOCTOR'S OFFICE!

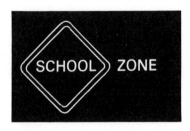

Keep learning everything you can from your doctor about diabetes and its treatment. He will also recommend reading material from a reliable source, such as, The American Diabetes Association.

You are learning when you make sure you understand the instructions your doctor gives you. If necessary, write them down while you are still in his office. Don't go home and wish you had.

You may not realize this, but with your doctor's help, your education on diabetes, is growing day by day!

Are you a regular reader of ADA FORECAST?

This bimonthly magazine is published by the American Diabetes Association, and written expressly for all diabetics, their families, and people around the world, in an effort to help everyone understand diabetes. It is indispensable as a source of learning.

Write to: American Diabetes Association, Inc.
           18 East 48th Street
           New York, New York 10017

1-2-3-4 TESTING LANE

Knowing "how" to test your urine specimen, and the "regularity" of testing, are extremely important, and fortunately, simple to do.

One of the chief complaints voiced by manufacturers and processors of testing equipment is, that the consumer does not read the instructions placed on the container. The user, often develops his own method of application, but when one's health and even life is involved, this can become a dangerous practice.

The urine test is the diabetic's only true indicator for control. He should read and follow the clear instructions, that come with the testing material.

Even a diabetic of long standing cannot determine his needs by "the way he feels" because the symptoms for both high and low blood sugar levels are many times similar, and a urine test is the only way to know.

Now, learning to test accurately and regularly is one of the first phases of control, your doctor will discuss with you. He will advise, what is right for you to use and how to use it.

Keep your testing equipment handy and always in adequate supply.

It is suggested by leading diabetic doctors, that one hour prior to the time of testing, the diabetic void, drink a glass of water and at the end of one hour, test the specimen. This test is made in one of two ways:

1. The "Tes-Tape" method is excellent for quick testing. Simply dip about 1½ inches of the tape, JUST ONCE, in the specimen, wait one minute and compare the color of the tape with the chart on the box. If the test shows ½ percent, then wait an additional minute, to see if it registers higher. Doctors tell us, to use the color at the end of the tape you are holding, for the true reading, as the color may vary.

While at home, practice the art of counting 60 seconds, so when you make tests away from home and do not have a second hand to watch, you will be familiar with the 60 second pace.

When using the Tes-Tape, don't waste it. It is so easy when in a hurry, not to wait the full one or two minutes, and risk not getting a true reading. You're wasting the tape. Worse than that, you are losing control of the diabetes and leaving yourself wide open for the development of infections, deterioration of blood vessels, and as a result, other parts of the body.

When you think of it this way, then it becomes easy to follow the instructions. You may find the cost of the tape is a little higher than the Clinitest tablets. However, the convenience, makes it popular.

2. Another test may be made with "Clinitest" tablets. Place five drops of urine and ten drops of water in the test tube (provided in the Clinitest kit), and add one Clinitest tablet. Wait until the boiling stops, then compare with the chart.

This is also an excellent time, while using the dropper, to make an "acetone" test. Place one drop of urine on an acetone tablet, wait one minute and compare with the chart.

It would appear that the Clinitest is less expensive, and perhaps even more accurate. However, it may be inconvenient to carry the kit for use away from home.

Both the Clinitest and Tes-Tape tests are hygienic, and there is no need to ever touch the specimen. Diabetics, doctors, nurses and technicians are grateful for both of them and their hygienic qualities.

It is known that a "zero" test and a "four-plus" are not completely measurable, but anything in between, is measurable. We don't know just how much "below" zero we are, nor how much "above" four-plus we may be, but we do know that too much in either direction is undesirable, and we should stay alerted for any possible emergency.

This testing knowledge can be applied to early detection of diabetic tendencies in all members of the diabetic's family. He should teach all members of the household to make these tests. Let's be alert to early detection of diabetes in our own family.

It is so easy to do.

REMEMBER THE CONTROL ADDRESS
1-2-3-4 TESTING LANE!

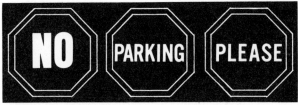

Being diabetic is no excuse for laziness, no more than it is an alibi for an acid disposition. The better the control, the more active the diabetic becomes, and—the happier he is! Physical activity burns up the unused sugar. When the diabetic feels the least like exercising, this may be the time he needs it the most.

A diabetic woman was taken to the hospital in a weakened condition. With the application of insulin and proper diet, she felt strength returning to her body.

As she was preparing to leave the hospital, she remarked to her doctor, "It is wonderful to feel stronger, will I now be able to do my own housework, like cooking, cleaning, washing and ironing? I just can't stand to be dependent upon other people any longer."

The doctor's reply was significant. "Yes, you will be able to do all of those things, and even more, if you abide by the simple rules." Thousands of diabetics have proved this to be true.

Of course, all things need to be done in moderation. Exercise, to the point of fatigue, can be harmful.

On one of Jolene's "better" days, she was trying to persuade her husband to permit her to mow the front lawn.

"The exercise and fresh air will do me good," she pointed out. Her husband was horrified and showed it.

"Why, you have NEVER mowed the lawn in the 20 years we have owned our own home! What would the neighbors think if I let you mow it now?"

"The neighbors don't bother me," Jolene answered. "Besides, I don't want to be a lily sitting on a lily pad. I want to help you do things, especially outdoors!"

Jolene knew his answer was final, but the never-give-up nature of a woman found her saying to her husband the next day, "Maybe I could mow the back lawn, not many neighbors would see me there."

Seeing the determination in his eyes, she continued, "You remember, I don't want to be — — —"

"I know," he broke in, "you don't want to be a frog on a lily pad." Jolene burst out laughing. "A LILY, not a frog." They both laughed.

Her husband won, by convincing her that there were many other satisfying things she could do, and still stay away from the easy life on a lily pad.

The diabetic woman's exercise is at her fingertips, right in her home. For the diabetic man, if his work does not include exercise, a brisk walk in the morning, and perhaps again in the evening, would be of real benefit.

Let's not be like the diabetic woman who felt so sorry for herself, she sat crumpled in a chair and "whined" about everything. Diabetics are not invalids. Don't let anyone wait on you. Insist on self-service. With control, you can be the king or the belle of the ball.

A controlled diabetic has a lot of energy, stored inside of him, and a great ability to express it.

SO, DON'T JUST PARK THERE, DO SOMETHING!

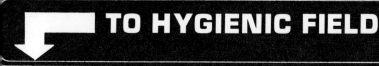

TO HYGIENIC FIELD

The diabetic has no choice, he NEEDS to be active in the hygienic field and be the cleanest person in the world!

Cleanliness is a "must" in every phase of diabetic living.

Start at the top. Keep your hair and scalp clean. This prevents infection of the scalp. When patronizing a beauty salon or barber shop, tell the owner and operator, that you are a diabetic.

Extra care is then taken to prevent burns, cuts, damage from bleaching, dyeing, et cetera. A woman would do well to purchase her own rollers, combs, nets, pins and whatever is used for the care of her hair, and carry them with her to the salon, each time.

The owner and operator will not be offended, but will understand the problem. Keep all articles clean and disinfected.

Next, fingernails should be kept short, clean and free from hangnails. If you show signs of allergy or sensitivity to nail polish or polish remover, like irritation of the skin, splitting, peeling or cracking of the nails, discontinue using them immediately. A manicurist should be told of the diabetic condition on the first visit.

A diabetic woman once said, "When I tell a manicurist I'm diabetic, I don't get a good manicure." Let's remember it is better to have a little less finesse, than no fingers.

Diabetes is relentless and often, we must back away from our wants, and be thankful for what we do get.

BY TRAVELING THE "EXTRA MILE" WITH CLEANLINESS, YOU GAIN MUCH BY EXPLORING AND WORKING IN THIS HYGIENIC FIELD.

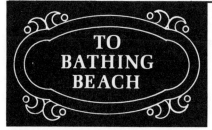

TO
BATHING
BEACH

The daily bath of the diabetic, is one of the most important parts of his routine. If each step is adhered to, many complications, both current and future, may be avoided.

This "daily" bath is necessary, for in addition to cleanliness, it stimulates circulation, kills and removes bacteria from the skin, reduces infections, and eliminates body odor.

When you are diabetic, care and caution must be exercised in many phases of the bath. It would be well to note several of them.

1. Because you should be relaxed and feel unhurried when taking your bath, choose a time when the bathroom is free (not when a line is forming outside the door).

Also, choose the time of day you are least likely to be sugar-free. Your balance, reflexes and coordination should be tops at that time.

2. Collect in advance everything you will need for your bath, like clean towels, washcloth, soaps, clean mat, clean clothes, creams and ointments. DO NOT SHARE ANY OF THESE ARTICLES WITH ANYONE.

3. Clean the tub well before using, and in addition, use one of the fine disinfectants for that purpose. If you find some cleaning preparation is making the tub slippery, then do not use it. Be sure to have permanent "non-skid strips" in the bottom of the tub.

A bar attached to the wall or the tub may be helpful when getting in and out. Use caution at all times. Never hurry with your bath.

4. It is extremely important that the water you draw, is not too hot. Doctors caution diabetics that the hand is not sensitive enough to test the water. The elbow should be used instead. If the water is too hot, burns could result. Testing the water takes such little effort.

5. It is an excellent idea to use a bacteria-killing deodorant soap. Permit it to remain on the skin for a few seconds before rinsing off. Then follow with your favorite fragrance soap, if you wish. You can kill the bacteria and still come out smelling like a rose. This gives you a double dividend—double cleanliness.

If you show tendencies of allergy to soap, or any bath preparation, be sure to seek your doctor's advice.

6. Step from the tub cautiously onto a clean mat or towel. (Be sure you have removed all bars of soap from the bottom of the tub.)

7. Freely apply one of the excellent antiseptic mouthwash/gargles, under the arms and in all crevices of the skin. This will kill any remaining bacteria on the skin and will reduce infections, boils, odor, itching and any other offensive problem of this type.

This suggestion was given Jolene Jordan about ten years ago by a nurse in the west. Since then, Jolene has not had another boil, itch or skin infection. Try it, you will like it too!

8. Sit down to dry yourself, another safety precaution. Apply a good ointment to your feet, as prescribed by your doctor. This will keep the skin pliable.

9. NEVER walk barefoot or with just socks on your feet. A sharp object on the floor can injure the foot. A stubbed toe can cause a lot of trouble, also. Wear clean "white" socks with bedroom slippers, for protection and cleanliness.

10. Use a good roll-on, spray or cream deodorant. If an irritation or itching appears as the result of its use, discontinue at once, and do not use again until you see your doctor. He will advise you on the brand most suitable for you.

Again, CAUTION is the watchword for every phase of the diabetic's bath.

A burn, or the broken arm or leg of a diabetic, may not heal as quickly as a non-diabetic's. It is still true, that—AN OUNCE OF PREVENTION IS WORTH A POUND OF CURE!

eye with caution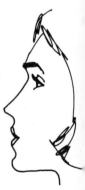

One of the most priceless possessions of mankind, his eyesight, is at stake after the onset of diabetes. Some diabetics experience problems early, while others live many years with the condition, before noting any changes in the eyes.

After 35 years of complicated diabetes, Jolene Jordan experienced several hemorrhages in one eye. As she sat in the office of an expert ophthalmologist, she heard him say, "You are what we call a victim of medical science."

Jolene said to the doctor, "Will it clear?"

He answered, "I don't know, we have to wait and see."

"If it does clear, how long will it take?" she asked.

"It's slow, maybe six months," he replied.

"Will it come again?" she pursued, almost fearfully.

"No one can say. I wish I could encourage you," he said.

Jolene is happy her eye did clear, and hopes with all her heart that even with the rapidly changing blood sugar she battles, it will not return.

Before insulin, diabetics did not live long enough to develop deterioration of the blood vessels which control the eyes. Here too, keeping the diabetes under control constantly, is one of the best preventions of blindness.

For the complicated diabetic, this may be a difficult procedure, for the rise and fall of the blood sugar is so extreme and rapid, that it is impossible to keep the urine free of sugar, every moment.

In such cases, doctors "may" recommend that some sugar show in the range of a trace, or a one.

AGAIN, BE SURE TO CHECK WITH YOUR DOCTOR.

This means that the complicated diabetic always carries the threat of eye hemorrhage, but this thought should urge him to work hard for the best possible control.

Any changes in the eyes should be reported at once to the diabetic doctor and the ophthalmologist. The wise diabetic has a yearly eye examination, whether he feels the need for it, or not.

SLOW DOWN ▶ DENTAL REPAIRS

Another sign on the dental road, says: Visit your dentist once every six months.

This is good advice for all people, but it is especially true for all diabetics.

Before insulin, the gums and teeth of the diabetic deteriorated rapidly, but now with good control, he can preserve them.

The diabetic should brush his teeth often every day, using dental floss and mouthwash for added protection. The gums should be carefully massaged after each brushing, stimulating circulation to the gums.

Since the diabetic does not eat sweets, he has the added benefit of preventing tooth decay.

This helps to slow down that dental repair job, and also, that repair bill.

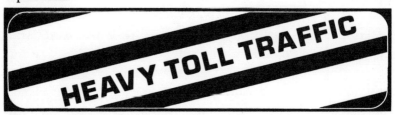

The battle of obesity is very real to the diabetic, for obesity is one of his worst enemies. Frequently it is the obese person who falls victim to diabetes, while his thinner brother or sister may escape.

When an obese person becomes diabetic, his doctor will immediately prescribe the loss of all excess weight. This helps to control the sugar, and the diabetic also discovers that he feels better, with the loss of each pound. This loss of weight often makes one more agile, active and alert.

Remember the selfish king who demanded the best food for himself, drank all the cream and gave the skimmed milk to his servants? The result? The king blubbered into a fat ball, while his servants became lean and strong. (We never found out if the king was diabetic.)

Recently, a very obese entertainer was seen on television partaking of food. Pressing it into his round jowls, said, "I like myself this way. Everywhere I go today, people are on a diet to lose weight. I can't stand people who are always on diets, and I don't want to talk about diets anymore."

When someone develops fat for fame and fortune, he is to be pitied. If padding his bank account is more important than health and appearance, that is his choice. Some day he may lie in a "too early" grave, and will have left a "fat" legacy for his heirs.

What happened to the jolly fat man, the whole world was supposed to love? Research tells us, this is a fallacy. The fat man was not really jolly, in fact, he was one of the most miserable creatures alive. And did the whole world love him? That's a question hard to answer. Maybe his mother did, but the rest felt sorry for him.

Certainly today, the fat man senses only pity, even ridicule, and the laughter he may inspire, may come from whatever entertainment he is providing.

A woman, who recently brought her weight down from 200 to 140 pounds, said, "I have just come to life. I have been sitting at home, so no one would see me, and now I can wear a playsuit and spend the afternoon in the park playing ball with the children. Everyone is happy, my children, my husband, but I'm the happiest of all!"

EVERYONE should keep his weight within normal limits, for when diabetes strikes, it usually chooses the obese person.

The organization TOPS (Take Off Pounds Sensibly) has as one of its slogans:

THERE IS NO FOOD WORTH BEING FAT FOR!

Obesity on the diabetic road, is bound to take its heavy toll.

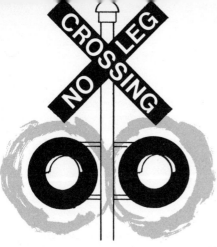

One of the humorous lines, universally experienced and understood, on which Pearl Bailey rose to fame, was, "My feet hurt."

The care of diabetic feet is extremely important, because the circulation of the blood to the extremities is often impaired.

Jolene sat in a class of diabetic patients, who were being taught the art of living normal lives in this new world of diabetic living.

She heard the teacher extol the importance of never "crossing" one's legs, since this habit can only impair the circulation of blood to and from the legs and feet.

This teaching might have been lost on Jolene, and perhaps on many other patients, except for the following incident.

Two days later, Jolene met some of her new diabetic friends under different circumstances in another waiting room.

The teacher of this previous day, walked into this same room, looked around, and—spotted an elderly gentleman, a Mr. Clark, with his "legs crossed."

Horrors of all horrors! The teacher embarrassed the gentleman in no uncertain terms, by reminding him of his forgetfulness of a previous lesson.

Jolene often remembered his embarrassment, but an important lesson was learned by every diabetic in that room. Mr. Clark, as well as everyone else who heard it, has probably never crossed his legs again.

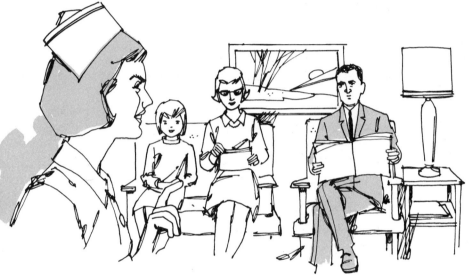

A rough lesson to learn, but who can say how many diabetic feet and legs have been spared from problems, and even amputation, through that one lesson, for no one in the room could have ever forgotten this rule and undoubtedly passed it on to many other diabetics.

Conscientious instructors are priceless, and this particular instructor was loved by all who came under her teaching.

There was a day when a visit to a podiatrist would have been considered the height of unnecessary expense and self-pampering. Today, his important role in promoting good health, is not challenged.

When the diabetic develops a foot problem, his doctor will invariably recommend a good podiatrist, and this is excellent.

A regular visit to his office, is a boon to everybody's well-being, but for the diabetic, it is imperative to his good health.

On your first visit to the podiatrist, tell him at once that you are diabetic. He will exercise special care, as he realizes that his usual cleanliness is very important.

A small blister or abrasion develops quickly, but heals slowly, or not at all. We are told some injuries respond to the wet treatment and some to the dry. The podiatrist recognizes this problem and applies the correct treatment at once. Don't delay. Procrastination in treatment can be disastrous.

Yes, the podiatrist is very important in the control of diabetes, and its complications. Diabetics everywhere, especially those who have watched his treatment and success in a minor or major problem, can sincerely say,

"HEAVEN BLESS THE PODIATRIST!"

A diabetic noticed a white fluid oozing from under a small callous below the large bone on his foot. After about a week of "hoping it would heal," he sought the help of his podiatrist who was shocked at the advancement of the abrasion, and asked, "why did you wait so long to see me? This is a pre-gangrenous ulcer, and no water must touch it for several weeks."

At the end of six weeks, after continuous treatment by the podiatrist, the foot was healed. The patient shudders to think what might have happened if he had not visited the able and informed podiatrist.

It is well to remember that any heating equipment, used by the diabetic, like hot water bottles, heating pads, heat lamps, et cetera, should be eyed with caution. If they are used on the feet and a burn occurs, many complications could follow.

Use this type of treatment only on the advice of your doctor. He will carefully inform you as to what precautions you must take.

Ask your podiatrist to recommend the type and size of shoes you require, and stay with his suggestions. Podiatrists tell us, many problems of the feet are caused by not wearing shoes wide enough.

The whole foot should rest on the sole of the shoe, not partly on the side of the shoe. Thick soles give the best protection, wedge heels for women, gives good support. This type of shoe helps prevent callouses, corns, irritated spots, et cetera. Several shoes, meeting this description, are on the market today.

Don't try to wear "old" shoes in the house, hoping to get by without blisters, abrasions or other complications of the feet. Be sure your "at home" shoes are just as well fitting as those you wear, to go out.

The same is true of bedroom slippers, and again, be reminded that it is a good idea to always protect the feet at home with clean white socks, and a diabetic NEVER walks barefoot or in his stocking feet. There is ALWAYS that danger of injury and infection.

Be sure the socks or hose you wear every day, are fresh and clean. It is a good idea to change your shoes two or three times daily. If one pair has a tendency to rub, a change in shoes will relieve the pressure.

The continuous use of adhesive tape on the feet is discouraged by podiatrists, as it may cause the skin to become tender and eventually, subject to open wounds. The diabetic should NEVER use adhesive tape on his feet, except under the direction of his podiatrist.

Of course, the diabetic NEVER uses corn removing ointments or liquids, or any other medication on his feet, without seeking the guidance of his podiatrist.

Discard at once, hose with holes or those that have been mended. It is easy to get into difficulty with a mended area, rubbing on the foot. Mending may delight the energetic and thrifty wife, but the result could be disastrous. The diabetic must realize he should never wear them.

There are those diabetics, who may not as yet have experienced problems with their feet, and therefore may not understand the seriousness of this warning.

Some may say, "It just couldn't happen to me." But those who have experienced it, know that diabetes plays no favorites, and that caution is better than correction.

Keeping the diabetes under the best possible control at all times, is the best prevention of deterioration of the blood vessels to the feet and legs, the onset of neuritis, infection, and yes, many other complications.

Let us not resent the precautions we must take. You have heard the story about the boy who complained when he had no shoes, until he met a boy who had no feet!

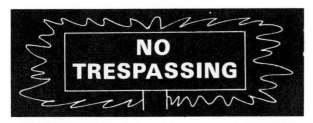

All diabetics have to learn how and when to say "No." Admittedly, this is not the easiest lesson to learn, but it is the first and most important step in getting and maintaining adequate control.

There are many occasions when diabetics meet head-on with the "No Trespassing" sign.

First of all, we must learn to say "No" to ourselves. Then it is easier to say "No" to our relatives and friends. The more experienced the diabetic becomes in control, the more he realizes the importance of this victory.

Some people feel that "going along with the crowd" is easier than saying "No." There is much room for doubt with this philosophy.

An insistent host or hostess may invite you to a party. To go, may be trespassing.

Or, if at the party, you may be urged to partake of refreshments. To do so, again may be trespassing.

In justification, you may say to yourself, adjustment in insulin and food can be made later. You may feel it more important to look and act like others. It is then that you are trespassing. You need to be strong. But, when declining, always explain your reasons.

One or two tries at the philosophy of "adjusting later" will convince you, this is wishful thinking. Persisting in this practice can only bring disastrous results.

It may be difficult to give up food and good times, but it is a challenge to the stability of every diabetic, and each time he wins, he senses strength, through better control. He is then, not a trespasser.

As family and friends become educated to diabetic living, they in turn, encourage the diabetic to maintain his control.

To insure a normal life for himself, his family and friends, the diabetic must pay attention to ALL of the road signs on the diabetic road, especially the one which has real meaning and purpose to him—

"NO TRESPASSING" PLEASE!

MERGING TRAFFIC

Merging our daily diabetic routine with the flow of our social activities, is something that must be done discreetly and planned well ahead.

By selecting wisely, it is possible for the diabetic to enjoy many wonderful occasions which were a part of his life, prior to the onset of this condition.

A diabetic woman attended a women's meeting, and it was her turn to "serve." Instead, she huddled in a chair, feeling very sorry for herself.

She felt too ill to do any work, so someone else took her place. BUT . . . when the cake was passed, she helped herself quite freely.

This weakness of character created a problem in three areas of her social world.

FIRST, because she allowed herself to get into this weakened condition, she was unable to take her place in the serving schedule.

If she was too ill to work, she was too ill to attend, and should have secured a substitute. Because of her lack of willpower she was sick and dejected and someone else had to do her work. How much better it would have been if she had been on the job, smiling, friendly and blooming with energy.

SECOND, she had so little control over her diet in public, she could not have had much at home. This kept her sick and in a weakened condition, necessitating the family, bearing the burden of her care. This is unfair.

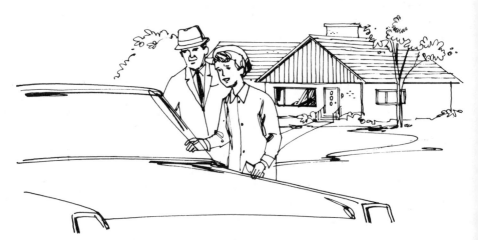

Enough misfortune can befall a controlled diabetic without hanging up a welcome sign for trouble. It takes real character to be a successful diabetic, so read and heed the road signs and you will avoid being a "drag" on anyone.

And in the THIRD place, she wasted the time of her doctor. After her "lunch" that day, she was so sick the following day, she had to use someone else's time to take her to the doctor, and rob him of some of his valuable time. Do you suppose she remembered to report the "extra" in her lunch?

The doctor is not a policeman, and has no desire to play this role. He can teach, warn, suggest and help the diabetic in many ways, but the diabetic must do the living.

This then, tells the story of what a diabetic should NOT do.

What should he do?

Each outside function needs to be considered on its own merit. Think first in terms of adequate diabetic control and then in terms of social obligations.

It is the deep desire of every diabetic to be active socially. But when he discovers that one activity brings on another, until the whirlwind of events prevents his keeping up with his control, he knows, decisions have to be made.

When his regular schedule is neglected, diabetic complications do set in. Soon he will get wise to this and put his diabetic schedule ahead of his social life.

The "stay at home" life is not advocated, nor completely necessary, but it is true, anything that interferes with daily control, should not be allowed.

"MERGING TRAFFIC" MEANS, A SOCIALLY BAL-
ANCED LIFE, BASED ON COMPLETE DIABETIC CON-
TROL!

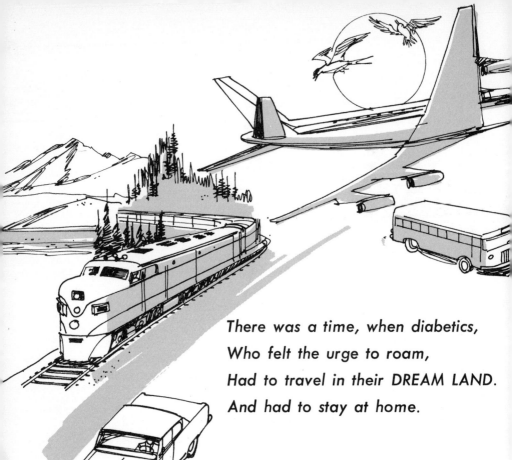

There was a time, when diabetics,
Who felt the urge to roam,
Had to travel in their DREAM LAND.
And had to stay at home.

With insulin, came freedom,
To travel far and wide.
Just like the other travelers,
Who take it all in stride.

So, AWAY WE GO, no matter where,
Without concern or care.
All diabetics travel well,
By land or sea or air.

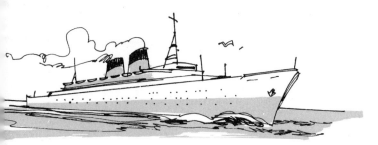

AWAY WE GO!

With the first breath of spring, the diabetic, like anyone else, feels the urge to travel.

Before the use of insulin, traveling could not be considered by the diabetic. Then followed a long period, when the advisability of it, was questioned.

Today, the diabetic has progressed in the understanding and application of his control, to the place where, fear for his health is gone. Now, he may feel free, to go on business trips or longed-for vacations.

Diabetic business executives, entertainers and leaders in many fields, who must travel, have become excellent examples of "people on the move."

Diabetes no longer hinders participation in the many modes of travel and pleasure.

There are, however, several considerations which help the diabetic to return home in as good a condition as when he left.

WHEN YOU FLY

It is the opinion of many in the know, that flying is the diabetic's best way to travel. The speed and comfort with which he arrives, is very beneficial.

Fifteen top airline companies were contacted by Jolene and asked the following questions:

1. What care do you provide for the traveling diabetic?

2. Do you have any recommendations as to what general slant or specific emphasis, might be directed to diabetics, as related to air travel?

The response from these companies was very gratifying. Their concern for and confidence in the traveling diabetic was heartwarming.

The general essence of their replies, was "Welcome aboard!" They had many helpful suggestions for the flying diabetic. Here are some of them.

Before you fly, ask your doctor for his approval.

If the doctor does approve, and has special instructions for the airline, he may call their office, and they will be happy to comply.

If you, the diabetic, know you need some special attention which only you, or someone in your family might recognize, then by all means take someone with you, who is capable of asking help in your behalf.

If your condition is critical, do NOT travel alone.

At the time the diabetic makes his reservation for the plane, tell the agent that you are diabetic, and ask for their special diabetic meal. This meal will be prepared in advance and placed on board, marked for the diabetic.

(Some companies serve diabetics the same meal as served to others, and expect the patient to use his judgment as to what he should eat.)

As soon as the diabetic is seated on the plane, he should immediately inform the stewardess of his condition, and identify himself as the one, who requested the special diet. Also, designate the time he would like the meal to be served.

When the stewardess is alerted to the fact that you are the diabetic, she will keep a "weather-eye" in your direction, in case you need help in any way.

Each company suggested that all diabetics who fly, keep themselves in good condition with adequate control, at all times. This responsibility, of course, is in the hands of the diabetic himself, and he must always be true to the trust.

Here, again, is another reminder, that the diabetic must AL-WAYS have with him:

Two bottles of each kind of insulin, or
Two separate containers of oral compounds
Two syringes
Two needles
Two Tes-Tapes
Adequate candy in some form

Disposable syringes and needles are excellent to use, when traveling. They are small and light in weight, always sterile and disposable on the spot. The needles, used only once, are never dull.

Small swabs of cotton soaked in alcohol and wrapped in aluminum foil, are also available. These supplies may be carried in pocket or purse, and are always ready for instant use. They do ease and simplify diabetic care. Many diabetics like to use these supplies at home, as well.

All letters from the airline companies were encouraging to the diabetic. Here are a few excerpts that may prove to be helpful.

One said, "There are no restrictions to air travel applicable to diabetics, provided they are under good control, are able to give themselves injections of insulin, if such is necessary, and understand the general diabetic treatment principles of their disease. We, like most major airlines, will supply special diabetic meals for such people."

Another company said, "Enclosed you will find a copy of the special meal request menus, including the diabetic meal. The meal is prepared, sugar free, and is available to any passenger requesting it, when reservations are made."

Other companies included with their replies, copies of pages from their Hostess Manual or treatment for diabetics in flight and material from their Flight Kitchen Manual, relative to special dietary requirements.

One of these letters read, "Because each diabetic has to know his own diet restrictions, we expect him to call and request his specific needs, as it would not be possible for any kitchen to prepare the meal to his total requirement, without advice relative to calorie intake, etc. In summary, it is our policy to provide any special diet requirement for any passenger, diabetic or other, who makes his requirement known."

The following letter seems to sum up the total coverage of all the problems a diabetic, a traveling companion, or stewardess, might encounter, while in flight.

"The carriage of diabetics as airline passengers have been performed for many years by the airlines without a great deal of inconvenience to either the passenger or the airline. The controlled diabetic falls into the category of an individual with a static illness who is ambulatory and is therefore acceptable under the criteria of passenger acceptance, accepted by all member airlines of the Air Traffic Conference of America. The diabetic who is brittle, poorly controlled, or who has an impending acidosis condition, is in a different category in that he is non-static but ambulatory and may have to receive a medical review before carriage, if this is necessary.

"We, therefore, feel in general that the controlled diabetic should present no problem to average air carriage by airlines.

"In my experience with relation to passenger comfort and discomfort aboard aircraft, which dates back to 1938, I would state unequivocally that, at the present time, and certainly within the last five years, we have had fewer and fewer problems with known diabetics aboard our aircraft. This situation has improved because people are cognizant of the problems, they carry proper identification, and in general they are under more well controlled medical care than they have been in the past."

These replies from airline companies, serve to impress each diabetic once more, with the obligation he carries, TO EVERY-ONE, to maintain good control.

These letters then, should cause each diabetic to courageously lift his head, and march forward in confidence.

Each company has indicated real understanding of the diabetic, and gives him the assurance that he is—

"WELCOME ABOARD!"

WHEN YOU RIDE

Train and bus travel calls for prior planning and the constant awareness that problems and unforeseen complications may occur. For example, bad weather, mechanical breakdowns, or the unexplained delays that busses and trains are sometimes prone to, can cause real problems for the unprepared diabetic.

The diabetic should always have a double supply of medication and equipment and when traveling, this becomes DOUBLY important.

Keep in mind that the choice of food may be limited on a train or in the restaurants where busses stop. It is suggested that during rest stops on a bus trip that the diabetic purchase an extra sandwich to carry with him—just in case.

Keep a supply of sugar lumps or candy in the event of a severe insulin reaction.

A breakdown on the train or bus, may cause delay and further complicate the schedule. The diabetic must be prepared to meet such emergencies.

It is always wise, whether the trip be short or long, to carry extra food. This food, would need to be the kind that doesn't spoil without refrigeration.

There is also the risk of "weather" being a threat to the diabetic. There have been repeated experiences of snowstorms blocking railroad tracks and highways, and the stranded diabetic on a stalled train or bus, could be in difficulty.

Here too, the DOUBLE supply of medication and equipment will enable him to survive for sometime, IF he has adequate food.

In general, short trips by train or bus, may not be a problem to the diabetic, when he makes the proper preparation for complete control. However, even on short trips, the diabetic must anticipate many possible delays which could interfere with his control.

"THINK AND PLAN, BEFORE YOU RIDE!"

WHEN YOU DRIVE

Next to flying, it would appear that driving a car is the best way to travel. The diabetic then has complete control over everything!

He is free to stop anytime he wishes, choose the restaurant he prefers and stay as long as he pleases.

On a long trip, he is free to end his driving day whenever he feels the need.

This freedom and relaxation during travel, helps the diabetic to maintain his control.

The ability to choose the best place to eat, is one of the most important factors in diabetic traveling.

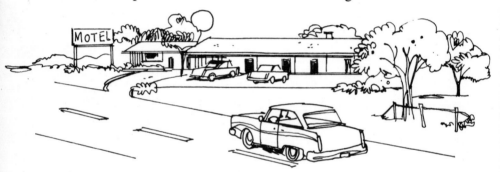

Since the public service personnel is not as yet completely educated to the diabetic's needs, it is difficult to obtain service exactly as needed.

All public eating houses would do well, to train their personnel in serving the diabetic, exactly as requested. The diabetic would then be happy to return for future meals.

Personnel should be taught, that when a diabetic identifies himself as such, and requests orange juice, or asks that his meal be served at once, he is not trying to wedge his way ahead of someone else.

No one need ever fear that a diabetic will exploit his condition to his advantage. There is something in the nature of a diabetic which makes him reluctant to ask for food. Everyone may be sure, when he seeks help, he needs it, and fast.

Each year, Jolene Jordan and her husband travel by auto to a city in the southwest. They take the same route each time, because they are acquainted with the habits of certain eating places, their hours of service, and their understanding of special needs.

Jolene says, they have found it to be important to drive only the required distance each day, to bring them to one of these better places. If restauranteurs understood this important consideration, they would bend every effort to meet the need.

There are additional reasons, why a diabetic needs to be careful, while traveling. Sometimes a change in climate, a change in food or drinking water, and adjusting to the gain or loss of one hour, when traveling from one time zone to another, all these may contribute to complications.

These are the reasons why doctors advise the traveling diabetic to watch his control carefully. Should he suspect an approaching problem, he should contact a local doctor at once.

When traveling by car, place an "ice chest" in the trunk, and keep several oranges ready for emergency use. You may never need them, but be prepared!

In order to keep a fresh supply, use some of the oranges for breakfast and desserts, but never let the supply run out. Don't use them and EXPECT to replace them later. Replace them FIRST!

Other foods that are not always obtainable in a restaurant, may also be kept in this ice chest. If you are in a warm climate and the weather is cooperative, a lunch at the roadside may be quite enjoyable.

If others in the party, prefer a restaurant, there should be no objection to the diabetic eating his food on time at the road-side. The fellow travelers may then feel more at ease, when being served later, in a restaurant.

When choosing a place to sleep, select the cleanest one you can find. The few extra dollars may be a good investment. When you check in, be SURE to ask for the correct time, as it may have changed, since you last set your watch. Also, in-quire what time the dining room opens the following morning. An injection of insulin and a closed dining room, present problems.

Several times, when Joan Crawford was interviewed on TV, she told of her interest in cleanliness in the overnight room assigned to her. Each time she visits a new room, her first act is to scrub EVERYTHING before using the room and bath. Many people, and certainly diabetics, share her feeling, and all people would do well to follow her example.

Here too, if motel and hotel management knew, how much this meant to ALL travelers, they would place greater em-phasis on cleanliness.

Yes, driving short or long distances, brings pleasure to all, but to the diabetic who has not always been able to enjoy this type of pleasure, it brings great delight, and public service em-ployees can help the diabetic in many ways to enjoy his travels from coast to coast.

CAMPS FOR DIABETIC CHILDREN

Sending a diabetic child to a summer camp, designed for diabetic children, is a wonderful way to help him learn to live a normal and happy life.

Here, he becomes acquainted with other children who are living with the same problems and restrictions. All are taught about their diabetic condition, the importance of care and attitude, the selection and preparation of their food, insulin, and how best to inject it.

They receive physical examinations which are always helpful, and they learn the general rules for living with their problems and the art of cooperation.

They receive all of this help and, at the same time, are enjoying the thrills of camplife and many other happy experiences.

Seek your doctor's advice, and if for any reason he feels your child should not go, he will tell you so. If he feels it is wise, he may wish to help you select the camp best suited to your child. He will also help you, regarding the contact with the camp officials, in case special help is needed.

A list of summer camps is available by writing the American Diabetes Association, 18 East 48th Street, New York, New York 10017.

Perhaps there is no better way, to help the diabetic child develop into a normal adulthood, than to expose him to the normal and happy association with children of his own age and style of living.

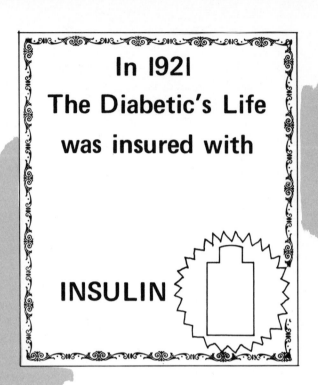

In 1921
The Diabetic's Life
was insured with

INSULIN

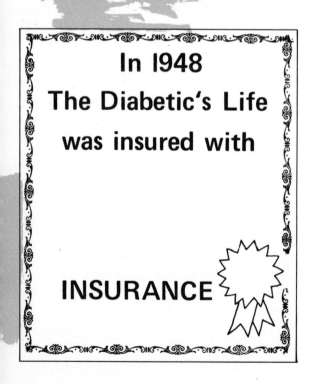

In 1948
The Diabetic's Life
was insured with

INSURANCE

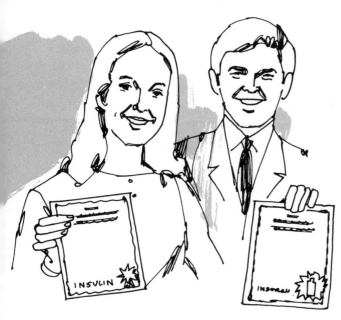

INSURANCE FOR THE DIABETIC

One of the greatest comforts offered to the controlled diabetic today, is the privilege of becoming an insurance policy holder. Up until about 20 years ago, the diabetic was uninsurable.

This one benefit alone, brings a new confidence, challenge, incentive and purpose to the controlled diabetic.

The security of being insured is a great reward for adherence to the rules of diabetic living. Any sacrifice or rigidity, experienced in his living, which might at times seem irksome, becomes a desirable way of life.

Those who live with and trust their future to the diabetic, sense this security also.

One of the questions insurance companies ask, is "WHO is a PREdiabetic?"

Diabetes may have been prevalent in the family, without the insured being aware of it. The insured's parents may have been carriers of the condition and could have passed it along.

The insured may be a carrier and some day pass it on to the next generation. But he could also develop the condition during his own lifetime, without knowing that anyone else in his family was diabetic.

These are a few of the reasons why insurance companies must question all potential policy holders concerning any known diabetic history in the family. They also need to know from which side, or whether from both sides of the family, victims of this condition appeared.

When you apply for insurance, be SURE to tell the company representative your full story. He will help you. You owe this honesty to him.

When the controlled diabetic IS insured, he owes his best self-care, not only to himself and to his family, but now also to the insurance company. He must prove himself worthy of those who have placed their confidence and faith in him.

The insurance companies are one of the best diabetic detection sources. Many insurance seekers, who are required to have physical check-ups before receiving insurance, have been discovered to have diabetes. Anyone detected in this manner, should be grateful.

There have often been discussions as to the advisability of a diabetic driving a car, because of the possibility of insulin shock, or any temporary imbalance which might affect his good judgment.

It is the consensus of opinion that each case must be decided on its own merit, and that the doctor is by far the best judge as to the severity of the illness, and if the patient's attitude and aptitude is such that driving is permissible.

Thousands of diabetics are driving cars every day. Insurance companies are not afraid to insure qualified diabetic drivers.

Thirty of the largest insurance companies in the United States, were asked' the following two questions by Jolene:

1. *What is your company policy as to limited or extensive coverage, extended to diabetics?*

2. *Would you have any recommendations as to what general slant or specific emphasis might be directed to diabetics as related to insurance?*

The replies came from the Medical Directors of each company, and indicated a sincere interest in adequate insurance for the diabetic.

Realizing how recently this confidence has been placed in the conscientious diabetic, the thrill of it, makes us tingle.

Here are a few sample excerpts from these letters. Be SURE to read them, and you too will understand better the problems, the solutions and the coverage, insurance companies offer today. Also, the important part every diabetic plays in obtaining adequate insurance.

"It is of interest to note that life insurance examinations are one of the foremost means of detecting unknown diabetics. Whenever this happens on a life insurance examination, we send a copy of the glucose tolerance test in a sealed envelope to the agency to give to the applicant for forwarding to his personal physician. . . . Within a matter of several months we are willing to review a report from the applicant's physician and if the diabetic situation is under good supervision and control, we are willing to accept the risk in accordance with our regular underwriting for diabetics."

"In a general way we take a liberal underwriting approach to diabetes which develops after age 50. This is usually a mild form and can frequently be controlled by dietary restriction and perhaps one of the oral hypoglycemic drugs. These cases we are willing to take at a low rating."

"While for a number of years the life insurance industry considered diabetics to be uninsurable at any price, experience has shown in recent years that many can be insured for a relatively small extra premium charge."

"I think another point worth mentioning with respect to insurance consideration, not only from our company practices, but from those of the industry, is that predicting a diabetic's life span of likely good health is influenced considerably by the condition of his circulatory system."

"Diabetics are not all alike. The only fair basis for insuring them is to view each on the merits of his individual situation."

And now, one more:

"The primary lines of insurance that come to mind as deserving some comment seem to be life insurance, disability insurance and perhaps automobile insurance. From an automobile insurance standpoint, there is no unusual problem that would face the diabetic as long as there is every indication that his condition is controlled. In a particularly difficult case, the issue might well be resolved by a physician's statement to the effect that, in the physician's opinion, the patient is or is not in a position to safely operate an automobile."

"To be insurable, a diabetic must have his condition under control. This is usually evidenced by the patient's cooperation with his doctor."

*   *   *   *   *   *   *   *

NOW, YOU KNOW! These letters are proof of what is expected from the diabetic by the insurance companies. It can be summed up, this way:

SEE YOUR DOCTOR REGULARLY, AND
MAINTAIN DAILY CONTROL!

If any diabetic has been unimpressed with the importance of adequate daily control, we hope he now realizes that his constant control is vital.

When insurance companies put such obvious emphasis and warning on control, it is time ALL diabetics recognize the risks of impending danger, and LIVE according to the doctor's guidance and advice daily!

The reward is rich and lasting. Follow these suggestions, because it involves YOUR success, YOUR health, YOUR life!

"LIFE INSURANCE DEPENDS ON YOU!"

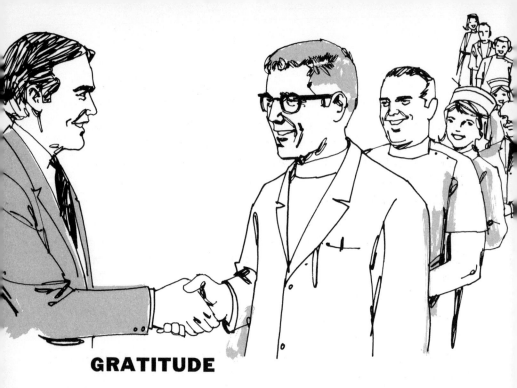

GRATITUDE

When anyone is told he is diabetic and must take insulin or an oral compound for as long as he lives, he is apt to drift into despondency, self-pity, or even despair.

However, as weeks and months pass by and improvements in his condition have taken place, he exchanges this despondency for courage, self-pity for happiness and despair for hope.

Quite suddenly the diabetic accepts the life-line of insulin with gratitude, and as a result, improves his attitude toward his condition.

As the diabetic once more finds himself able to do his work, he assumes his old responsibilities and once more enjoys his family and friends. As he reminisces and compares what he was with what he is now, his gratitude continues to increase.

If each diabetic were to make up his own list of people who have helped him in adjusting to diabetic living, he would come up with an impressive list.

Each patient would include in this list, many doctors, nurses, family members and friends. However, each one, without exception would also head his list, with the names of two men who have given all diabetics, not only hope instead of despair, but also life instead of death.

The whole world knows these men to be Dr. Frederick Grant Banting and Dr. Charles Herbert Best, co-discoverers of insulin.

During their days of research, they endured and surmounted obstacles, failures, disappointments and even antagonism. However, their perseverance won, and they gave the world insulin, with new hope and life for the diabetic.

Dr. Banting's work was cut short during World War II, when he lost his life in a plane crash in Newfoundland, while doing research for the Canadian government.

Dr. Best is presently Director of Research at Toronto University, Toronto, Ontario. He has continued his work relentlessly, through these many years. His research might some day reveal the cause and cure of diabetes. For this hope, diabetics are also grateful.

Before Dr. Banting died, he is reported to have said, "Not one diabetic ever wrote to thank me for insulin." Diabetics, like other patients, so often are thoughtless. The desire for survival, causes a person to reach out for that proverbial straw, without a thought of what someone else might have to do, to provide that straw.

It is well for the diabetic to reflect on the days "before" insulin. At that time, each diabetic's diagnosis was scheduled to be an early statistic.

So great is the gift of insulin, which today provides a full life in place of a bare existence, that gratitude should grow day by day.

▶ IN BEHALF OF ALL THE DIABETICS, WE THANK YOU, DR. BANTING AND DR. BEST!

The diabetic's own doctor is so important to the continued well-being of the diabetic, that a schedule of contact is advisable. Many of the complications that are puzzles to the patient, are simple to answer for the dedicated diabetic doctor. Every diabetic should appreciate this help and guidance.

To all the doctors who direct and maintain the diabetic's health, day by day, we say, "Thank you!"

Thousands of diabetics are alive today, because of doctors' assistants, such as interns, nurses, aids, lab technicians and dieticians, who are also devoted to their duties. They have often helped to bring diabetics through difficult days of coma, complications, insulin reactions and many hospitalizations.

Each member of the hospital staff, also plays an important part in the recovery and sustained living programs of the successful diabetic. "Yes, we thank each one of you as well."

Every diabetic is grateful to his family and friends, for their respective contribution to his controlled and happy diabetic living.

Jolene Jordan knows what it has meant through the years, to have an understanding and helpful husband. Recently, a leading doctor in a large clinic said, "Jolene, I fully believe you have been helped greatly, and have found success in your diabetic living, because of the help of your husband." He spoke the words that Jolene has always known, and she replied, "Yes, you are right, more right than you even know."

Each diabetic needs someone to understand his problems better than anyone else, and help him each day, to hurdle the humps.

So, last but not least, for family and friends, we are truly grateful.

Therefore, in this spirit of appreciation, we say:

As gratitude now stirs our heart
And grows from day to day,
We want to show this gratitude
By helping OTHERS find their way.
For ALL of us need one by one
Live happily, from sun to sun.
Each night, let's feel that we have run
The race with courage and—have won.

With Jolene Jordan, now we say,

"GOD BLESS YOU, EVERYONE!"

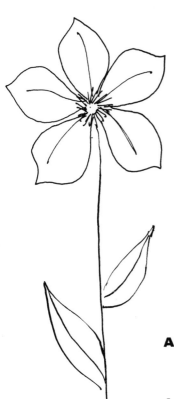

A PROMISE TO MYSELF

I pledge to live from day to day
In such a conscientious way,
That I shall be a diabetic
Who's well controlled and energetic.

SIGNED _____

HEREDITY

The following quotation on heredity appeared in the "FACT SHEET ON DIABETES" published recently by the American Diabetes Association:

Heredity and Diabetes

Diabetes is known to "run in families." The American Diabetes Association has estimated that as many as 50,000,000 or one out of four people may be "carriers"—that is, they may transmit diabetes to their offspring though most of the carriers will not develop diabetes themselves. Analysis of the Census survey by the National Center for Health Statistics[1] confirmed that diabetes does indeed "run in families" but that it may skip a generation or more. In only one percent of the diabetic population has diabetes occurred in three successive generations. One out of six had diabetic mothers and one out of twelve had diabetic fathers. But a majority knew of at least one diabetic parent or grandparent. One out of four of those with brothers or sisters knew of at least one brother or sister who also had diabetes.

[1]Public Health Service Publication No. 1000—Series 10—No. 40, Superintendent of Documents, U.S. Govt. Printing Office, Washington, D.C., August 1967.

A DIABETIC TRAGEDY!

A woman told of her mother refusing to take insulin, and that the oral products were ineffective. "How can we help her?" was the woman's question.

Anyone who needs insulin and refuses to take it, is a very selfish person. He is inviting trouble, and has not progressed far enough to realize the consequences of such neglect.

Everyone acquainted with the havoc, wrought by uncontrolled sugar in the system, knows it to be the forerunner of gangrene (a lost foot), blindness (helpless), a stroke (bedridden) and many more undesirable complications.

This woman's mother was inviting tragedy, not only for herself, but her family also. She should have asked herself, "Who will take care of me, should one or more of these handicaps befall me?"

Can there possibly be a woman, or man, or child in the world as selfish as this? There must be, for this story is true.

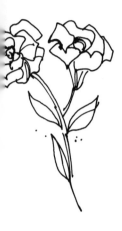

WHAT ABOUT CRASH DIETS?

Self-imposed crash diets for the purpose of losing weight, must never be a part of diabetic living. The American Medical Association recently said:

"The treatment of obesity cannot be isolated from concern for coexisting diseases such as diabetes and heart diseases, and requires very definite diagnostic skills and close supervision of the patient. . . . There are health hazards in weight reduction, and these should be thoroly understood and appreciated."

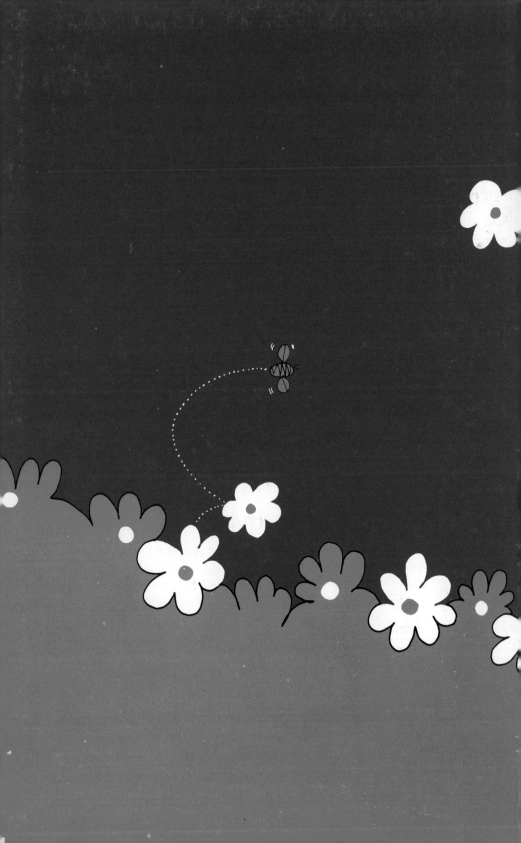